Better Brain Health

The Key to Your Six Cognitive Domains

John H. Dougherty Jr., MD

Medical Director of the Cole Neuroscience Center
University of Tennessee Medical Center

Interior layout by Robin Krauss, Book Formatters, www.bookformatters.com

Table of Contents

Preface

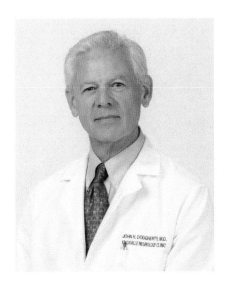

This is the 2nd Edition of our Better Brain Health guide. Dr. Dougherty, Andrew Dougherty and Sue Halliday have continued to assemble and update the latest information on prevention, treatment and overall brain health. This book will give you insight into aging, cognitive impairment and dementia, risk factors and how a brain healthy lifestyle can affect your cognition.

Everyone's brain works differently. We have our strengths and weaknesses, therefore our unique approach to improving your brain health focuses on all 6 cognitive domains. Using this approach we help you create a personal plan focused on achieving optimal brain health.

Throughout this book we will reference the COGselftest, which is an on-line screening tool developed to test each cognitive domain. You do not have to take the COGselftest in order to create your personal plan for a healthy brain.

You can't pick up a print newspaper or magazine, peruse on-line publications, review healthcare related blogs or watch national and local newscasts without the mention of memory loss, dementia, Alzheimer's disease and the importance of brain health. Of all the life-threatening health issues, individuals are most concerned about Alzheimer's disease. A new survey by the Marist Institute of Public Opinion found that regardless of age, Alzheimer's was the most feared disease – more than cancer, stroke, heart disease or diabetes. Our goal is to provide you with information that will help reduce the anxiety associated with aging and cognitive changes.

Of all the life-threatening health issues people face, Alzheimer's disease is the most feared. A new survey by the Marist Institute of Public Opinion found that regardless of age, Alzheimer's was the most feared – more than cancer, stroke, heart disease or diabetes.

The number one risk factor for dementia is age. Therefore based purely on the aging population, the number of individuals with dementia is going to rapidly increase. Of equal importance, the overall quality of healthcare is allowing us to live longer. These two factors, age and increased life expectancy, are contributing to the dementia epidemic.

Caring for your brain is as vital as taking care of your physical fitness, especially as you age. Did you know that an estimated 5.4 million people in the United States and 36 million people globally are living with Alzheimer's disease? Roughly 1.3 million people worldwide have early onset Alzheimer's. (before age 60)

Here are some sobering facts:*
- Alzheimer's disease was first reported by Dr. Alois Alzheimer in 1906
- Every 67 seconds someone in United States develops Alzheimer's disease (AD).
- More than 15.5 million people in U.S. provide unpaid care to those with AD.
- About 60 percent of those with AD go undiagnosed until it's too late in the disease for effective treatment.
- Alzheimer's is the 6th leading cause of death across all ages in the U.S. Recent data suggests Alzheimer's may be the 3rd leading cause of death.
- Among those Americans aged 65 & over with Alzheimer's, nearly 2/3 are women.
- One in three older adults die with Alzheimer's or another form of dementia.
- The annual cost of care for Alzheimer's disease is over $210 billion in the U.S. and is expected to rise to $1.2 trillion by 2050.
- Women in their 60s are almost twice as likely to develop Alzheimer's over the rest of their life as they are to develop breast cancer.
- Of all the people who ever lived to be 65 in the history of the world, 2/3 are alive today.

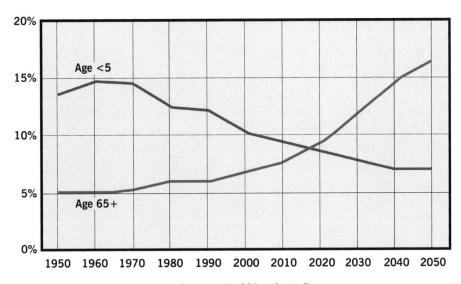

Source: United Nations World Population Prospects

In the past we didn't understand the impact of environmental factors such as physical and mental exercise, nutrition, stress, socialization and education on our brain health.

We started writing this book and developing the COGselftest because we knew we needed to do something to stem the tide of the coming epidemic that is increasing the incidence of Alzheimer's disease. We can only do that through education, early screening, intervention and awareness.

The COGselftest, which was first developed in 2007, is now available to everyone. Initially, the development of an online self-test was focused on patients with Alzheimer's, but it was necessary for us to make modifications for it to truly be comprehensive. It tracks various types and degrees of cognitive impairment in each of the six cognitive domains of the brain. The patterns shown in the results of the test offer those who take it the possibility of identifying cognitive changes that could be associated with Alzheimer's or other forms of dementia earlier.

Of course, the software aspect of the COGselftest is not the end of the story. We took the time when we were developing the test to validate the test scientifically. The COGselftest was compared to existing tests to show its benefit. All of this took a tremendous amount of time and effort, and continues to this day. Subsequently, the COGselftest analysis results were published in the Journal of Alzheimer's Disease—which is peer-reviewed. The COGselftest showed a 96% accuracy rate in a random sample, and a 93% accuracy rate in classifying Alzheimer's disease and cognitive-impaired groups.

This kind of online test is more important than ever before, especially after

Medicare's announcement that beginning January 1, 2011, all beneficiaries are required to be screened for cognitive changes as part of their Annual Wellness Visit (AWV).

Although in the health care industry requirements may change, you can be confident that getting results from the COGselftest will empower you to take charge of your brain health.

The COGselftest provides an alternative to traditional paper-based methods for assessing neurobehavioral and cognitive functions. An individual can complete the COGselftest alone or with a caregiver or family member who can facilitate interfacing with the computer.

The COGselftest is a screening tool for evaluating all 6 cognitive domains and is not in and of itself a diagnostic measure for cognitive impairment.

I hope you enjoy this book. We have tried to give you a common sense approach to the way your brain functions and outline what you should do to further improve your brain health.

Sincerely,

John H. Dougherty, Jr., MD Knoxville, January 2015
(Association, 2014)

In Appreciation

It is true that in writing this book, I have become wiser from advice received from expert colleagues. Aided by hundreds of specialists in neurology, along with over 3,000 patients, I believe that Better Brain Health will become a practical resource—which I alone could not have written. I wish to thank some key health information experts, without whom this book would not have been written:

Sue Buckley Halliday – Her experience as the founder of AHRMemory and co-founder of MI-COG, LLC, which offers news and resources on brain health, early memory loss and dementia—has been extremely valuable. Ms. Halliday's expertise in PET/CT imaging, as well as her knowledge of medical policy development, helped immensely in examining all angles of brain health. Finally, her advocacy for those seeking guidance about early memory loss and dementia has been inspiring.

Ruth Tesar – As CEO of Northern California PET Imaging Center and co-founder of MI-COG, LLC, Ms. Tesar is working on a public-private partnership that will bring a new PET radiopharmaceutical research lab to Sacramento. Through such efforts, she aims to advance clinical care in specialties such as oncology, cardiology and neurology. Her knowledge of healthcare policy also is invaluable, as she has played a role in obtaining coverage for PET procedures from private payers and the Centers for Medicare and Medicaid Services.

Finally, I'd like to thank my son **Andrew Dougherty**, who is Co-founder and President of Medinteract. We started this journey together in 2004 and seeing his passion and expertise about AD has truly been one of the great experiences of my life. I am extremely proud of how he has become a well-known authority on brain health information, and am so grateful for his support.

My gratitude extends to colleagues who have contributed medical, healthcare, and communications advice for this book. For their encouragement, wisdom, and time, I also thank the people named below:

Walker Buckley, Chief Development Officer, MI-COG, LLC (CognitiveTest. com)

Laura Carlson, Founder/Sr. Writer, Alpha Marketing

When the original book was released for publication, I began gathering more information for this second edition. Your input will influence how this book will evolve over the years. So please feel free to share your thoughts at betterbrain@ medinteract.com.

Medical Interactive Education, LLC
106 W. Summit Hill Dr. Suite 301
Knoxville, TN 37902

Andrew's Personal Story

Perspective on a relative with Alzheimer's

My grandmother Florence Dougherty was a most amazing woman. She was director of the Women's Job Corps in Knoxville, Tennessee during the Civil Rights movement. I believed she was indestructible.

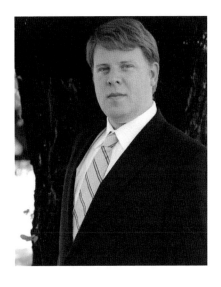

But by 1986, at the age of 72, she began to show signs of dementia. Back then, little was known about mild cognitive impairment (MCI). It is a precursor to Alzheimer's disease and doesn't affect the activities of daily living. My grandmother probably had MCI for at least eight years before it progressed to early Alzheimer's. She had an atypical form of AD in which the progression is very slow.

One of my first realizations that something was amiss with my grandmother's mind was when I was about six years old. My dad and I had discovered a chipmunk that had been injured and took it back to her house to nurse it back to health. At that point, my grandmother was confused on who we were and what we were doing. She remembered my dad—although she did not recall his name. She might not have known who I was, but she knew that I belonged there with her.

The next memory that resonates with me was when our family was visiting grandmother in the nursing home. At that time, I was perhaps 12 or 13. My grandfather had brought a gift of Russell Stover chocolates to my grandmother. These candies were her favorite, but she was not aware of who he was, or who my parents and I were. What I remember most about that visit was that my grandmother was speaking only in French. I believe she had studied French when she was younger, and perhaps the part of her brain that stores the knowledge of language had the least amount of atrophy. My takeaway from that experience was that the brain is an amazing organ with immense power—I am not sure if it will ever be fully understood on a scientific and emotional level.

I often wondered whether my father (Dr. John Dougherty, Jr.) became a neurologist in part because of his mother or if it was purely his fascination with the brain. He started his focus on AD in the last 18 years, although it is my belief that it had always been something that interested him. In 1984, he was instrumental in establishing the Cole Neuroscience Center at the University of Tennessee Medical Center, and a year later was elected to the first board of the Alzheimer's Association in Knoxville. I believe that even then—almost 30 years ago—subconsciously, he realized that AD would become one of the most prominent diseases of the next generation. While the world was tackling AIDS and cancer, the population of "Baby Boomers" was getting older and their life expectancies were increasing, which compounds the major risk factor for AD—age.

My first in-depth experience with AD was volunteering at an adult day center run by the organization now known as Alzheimer's Tennessee when I was 13. At the time, I did not understand the full ramifications or effects that the experience would have on me, but I saw the challenges facing caregivers, and many of these obstacles still remain today.

My lasting impression of that experience was of one particular patient who was an ex-Navy boxer. When he became confused and frustrated he would take his clothes off and try to box the caregivers or other patients. At that time, it was both a humorous and depressing experience for me—but it emphasized how powerful and important the brain is to our bodies. At 19 I worked in a brain bank, a collaboration between Alzheimer's Tennessee and the University of Tennessee, where we dissected brains and looked at the epidemiology behind the plaques in AD. I went on to receive a BSM in finance and information systems from Tulane University. I was drawn to technology and the rapid rise of the Internet, so I went to work at a start-up online travel company in Atlanta, GA.

During that time, I had a phone conversation with my father in which he told me something that literally changed my life. At this point his primary focus was Alzheimer's disease and he realized that the major problem was a lack of education. He said, "It might be that we [neurologists] have not done a good enough job yet in educating the medical community and laypersons about Alzheimer's disease."

I decided to come back to Knoxville and see if I could work with my father to make an impact on this omission in education. In 2004, we formed Medical Interactive Education, LLC with a mission to spread knowledge about cognitive issues ranging from diagnosis to treatment. From a business perspective and technology background, I saw the opportunity in web-based interactive seminars.

Selling my car for the initial startup money, I decided that the best way to reach the physicians and generate revenues was through the pharmaceutical companies and their representatives who are in front of physicians and have a monetary incentive to educate them. My dad and I introduced online training courses to pharmaceutical representatives, and physicians across the country. However, the trend at that time was toward physician-to-physician talks. The problem was this: How can we give primary care physicians the incentive to learn about AD and its diagnosis? We simply did not have the resources, experience and time to reach our audience and make it fiscally possible.

I concluded that to become successful in achieving this goal, I needed to learn more about business and received my MBA from the University of Tennessee with concentrations in finance and entrepreneurship/innovation. I worked as an analyst for a venture capital firm and got valuable experience in startups, business strategy, marketing, fundraising, and financial analysis amongst many other business activities.

In further discussions with my father, we determined that the first problem we needed to solve was the diagnosis of AD. The statistics were staggering— that 60% of AD cases are not diagnosed; and in those cases that were diagnosed, it was usually too late for effective treatment options.

I am often asked why I did not pursue a career in medicine like my father, grandfathers, and mother—who are all in the medical field. My answer is that I realized the way to make a substantial impact in healthcare involves not just the knowledge and impact of a physician and researcher, but also the business and financial expertise that is necessary for innovation. With the combination of neuroscience and entrepreneurship, I believe we can make a great contribution toward the wellbeing of future generations—of providing vital information, diagnosis and treatment for AD and various forms of dementia.

__Andrew I. Dougherty, MBA__
Medinteract, President

CHAPTER 1

Understanding Your Brain

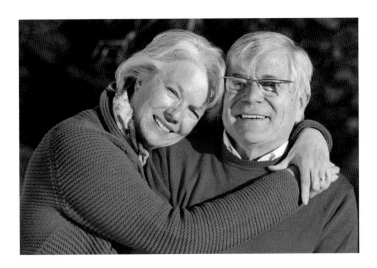

The brain is a fascinating, complex organ. It has the amazing ability to reason, perceive and store memories. To protect this brainpower, it's helpful to understand more about human "cognition." Basically, it's the process of acquiring and comprehending knowledge through our senses and experiences.

The overall spectrum of cognition includes three categories: Normal Aging, Mild Cognitive Impairment and Dementia.

Normal Aging

As recently as 15 years ago, the concept of "senility" was commonly used to describe the normal aging process. For example, the prevalent thought was that it is a part of normal aging for our grandparents to forget our names. We now know that this concept is outdated and incorrect.

As we age, it is common to experience some decline in processing and recall of new information. Things might become slower or it might be more difficult to remember names or follow instructions on your new mobile phone. Have you ever forgotten where you parked coming out of the grocery store or have you ever been talking on your phone while looking for your phone? The good news is that this is completely normal! The brain interprets millions of sensory inputs every minute and people categorize those in different ways. Depending on your ability to focus, certain tasks are easier to perform or recall than others.

Dr. Dougherty describes a situation with someone worried about her memory. "I had one patient come into the office complaining that she was forgetting everything and was sure that she had early Alzheimer's disease. After testing and examination, the results were that she was completely normal. She took out her iPhone and pulled up her calendar to show me how she was missing appointments and forgetting contact phone numbers. After a few minutes spent going through her phone she realized that she was not saving the appointments on her phone, but only on her computer. This is an extreme example, but it shows us how we can become consumed with our worries of Alzheimer's and start to believe that we have problems when they do not exist."

The normal aging process includes some brain atrophy, which is shrinking of the brain caused by the loss of cells. On average, the brain shrinks by about 1.9% every 10 years. This shrinkage increases every year after the age of 60. As scary as this seems, it does not mean that people lose cognition or overall brain function. It just means that the brain might not be as efficient in getting the job done. Abnormal brain atrophy can be caused by dementia, seizures, traumatic brain injury or difficulty with language. The good news is that in many cases we can prevent or slow the progression of brain atrophy through exercise and nutrition, which we detail in later sections of this book.

Mild Cognitive Impairment

The term "Mild Cognitive Impairment" (MCI) describes early problems with cognitive function. By definition, MCI includes impairment usually in a single cognitive domain, is insidious in onset (proceeding in a gradual, subtle way) but does not impair social or professional skills. The most common domain affected is memory. This does not mean that a person with MCI cannot function regularly in their daily life. And a diagnosis of MCI does not necessarily mean that one will progress to AD. In fact, some people with MCI can revert back to normal while others might stay in that classification throughout their lives. In my family, the progression from MCI to AD lasted about eight years.

"I have several patients diagnosed with MCI who are still active in their professions of business, law and medicine."
– *Dr. Dougherty*

There are two types of MCI:
1. **Amnestic** – This is the most common form and
   it affects memory. Typically 8 to 10% of those with amnestic MCI
   convert to AD each year.

2. **Non-amnestic** – This kind of MCI usually affects verbal fluency, the ability to create language, and 15 to 20% of these convert to dementia each year.

While 8 to 10% of individuals diagnosed with MCI convert to Alzheimer's disease (AD) within one year, 20% of individuals revert to normal within one year. So a diagnosis of MCI is not a cause for panic so much as it is a call to action. MCI can be caused by a number of things and sometimes it can be difficult to track down these causes. However, studies of individuals with MCI who take Cholinesterase Inhibitors (CEIs) such as Aracept have shown a slower rate of conversion to AD, usually 12 to 24 months slower.

Although there have been some mixed study results on the use of CEIs, the most recent study in the New England Journal of Medicine provides support for CEI effectiveness up to 24 months. Your physician may prescribe CEIs for MCI and watch for results.

What does the term BIOMARKER mean?

A biomarker is something in the body that can be measured and reliably indicates the presence or absence of disease or the risk of later developing a disease. For example, your blood sugar level is a biomarker for diabetes or your cholesterol level is a biomarker for heart disease. Cognitive tests, MRI and PET scans are a few of the biomarkers for dementia.

Prodromal Alzheimer's Dementia

The term "prodromal" Alzheimer's dementia is used to distinguish individuals diagnosed with MCI who also have one or more positive biomarkers associated with the neuropathology of Alzheimer's disease.

Understanding Early Warning Signs

This section discusses some of the most common symptoms associated with cognitive changes.

Repeated and persistent signs of forgetfulness

As people age they frequently complain of losing keys, misplacing a wallet, purse or checkbook, or some other staple item. With normal aging you may forget where you parked your car after shopping, or you may forget a turn or two in the car but not actually be lost. You may even go to the pantry, only to forget what you went for, but you can retrace your steps or think for a moment and recall. The concept of forgetting briefly but then being able to reason out a way to the memory in the mind is very normal.

This is not so for people with Alzheimer's disease (AD). Someone with

AD may be incapable of remembering where the car is parked, or may find themselves driving with no idea where they are or how to navigate from there. The inability to eventually pull out the recent memory is not normal.

Diminishing success using everyday items

People with AD frequently have trouble operating a microwave, not just adding 30 second increments, but may have lost the ability to set cook time and power or program the defrost mode. They may also have trouble using kitchen utensils or everyday tools, especially individuals who typically perform household projects with ease.

Someone with worsening symptoms may be putting clean dishes away and have trouble recalling where the dishes are supposed to go. They may also have a difficult time getting the dishes put in the right place. Another example would be an individual washing the same load of clothes over and over.

Memory problems

Problems with memory deficits tend to worsen over the course of a year or so, which is a very typical progression for AD. After one year there is often more difficulty with recent memory and recalling conversations, trouble remembering to tell someone of a phone message they took for them, or to recall what was discussed in a call they just completed. Recent memories are the key here. Past memories may be fully intact for people with AD. They may have no idea what they ate for breakfast but will be able to recount early times in their lives with ease. Anxiety over memory loss can exacerbate these problems.

Word recall

People in the slow progression of cognitive decline often have trouble recalling every day words or have difficulty selecting the right word to use.

One who is experiencing normal aging may see a clock on the wall and recognize that it has hands and numbers, but momentarily lose the word clock. The word clock will eventually come to them. Individuals may forget the names of people they do not see on a regular basis – this can be completely normal.

People with AD have trouble recalling the names of people they do see regularly. They may not be able to eventually pull the word clock out of their memory, no matter how well they can describe the device itself. As mentioned above, anxiety over this issue can be an extenuating factor.

Now we will look in more detail at areas in your daily life where symptoms of early AD may appear. This will help you better distinguish normal aging from the signs of something more serious.

Other symptoms and potential warning areas for people with early AD

Many people with early AD will have trouble with processing tasks such as the ability to balance a checkbook, pay bills or cook meals. It is important to delineate between cooking something simple and planning and cooking a full meal. Pulling together an entire meal is usually much harder for someone with AD.

Handling cash, making change and calculating the tip in a restaurant are examples of everyday processing tasks with which people suffer in early AD. Driving can also be affected and it is important to monitor driving skills first hand and understand their ability to control the car and abide by the legal speed limit. Watch for driving too slow and keeping the car within their designated lane.

Specifically, have they gotten lost while driving? One problem facing individuals with AD is they can generally operate their vehicle but often experience significant visual-spatial impairment. This leads to people going the wrong direction on a one-way street, reacting to a red light by stopping far back from the intersection or bumping the curb while trying to navigate a turn.

Other symptoms to look for in the home include using the TV remote, not just the ability to turn it on or off, but do they go into the listing guide and select the station they want to watch from the list? Do they safely use the microwave, not just start and stop but programming tasks like thawing or using other settings? The same concern would apply to the stove – can they cook without burning the food, do they remember to turn off the burner and can they use pre-heat and timed cook settings on the oven?

Even with relatively early AD people will remember who is associated with their speed dial settings. Many older adults are computer literate. For these individuals – are they able to send emails and can they search the web successfully, as this is a difficult task requiring use of multiple programs?

Evaluation of a new patient by Dr. Dougherty

When I'm evaluating a new patient I try to see if I can develop a scenario of progressive worsening over time. Perhaps two years ago they were experiencing symptoms of forgetfulness and then one year ago they began to repeat themselves, asking the same questions, for example, even when they have already received an answer. This is a typical progression for AD.

I always ask if they have difficulty with balance or coordination, problems with bladder or bowel control or gait disorders. These can be signs of vascular dementia, not AD, so it's important to differentiate between types of dementias as early as possible.

Early Alzheimer's or Depression?

Twenty percent of people with AD also develop depression, so it is not uncommon for a person with AD to also be depressed. During an initial consultation an individual can show characteristics of AD, however, after a thorough evaluation there are no clinical signs of AD and a diagnosis of depression is made. So an individual could show apparent symptoms of AD and be in one of following groups:

1. They actually have AD
2. They have both AD and are depressed
3. They are experiencing pure depression with no associated AD.

This is a crucial distinction. If symptoms are present it is important to have a physician conduct a full evaluation, since making the clinical determination can be difficult.

One unique way we can address this challenge is through associated memory. Here's something you can try at home: ask the individual to remember 3 words, for example telephone, police, river. Have them repeat the words aloud to you and then go back to whatever they were doing. Wait 10 minutes before asking them to repeat the words.

This is free recall – asking them to repeat the words with no help from you. If they cannot remember all 3 words then give them a clue or a bit of information to help them identify the category, without giving away the word. For example, if they miss the word "phone" you might say: one word I asked you to remember is a means of communication.

A patient who is depressed will find the clues very helpful and be able to recall all three words. This associated recall will not, however, help a person with AD. The words will be irretrievably lost. The defect here is in the hippocampus and temporal lobe, which prevented the individual from laying down new memories when they heard the words initially.

With pure depression, the memory is laid down but the depression itself causes an "attentional" defect. The inability to pay complete attention initially interferes with memory of the words during free recall. Since the memory was initially laid down however, the clues will help depressed individuals to retrieve the words.

This is another example why taking a thorough history can be very helpful at distinguishing early AD from other problems which may present with similar symptoms.

Dr. Dougherty discusses driving

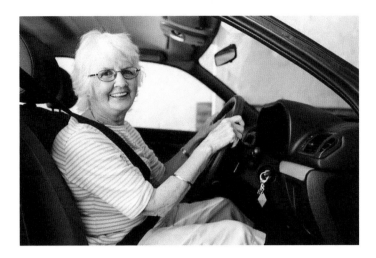

The caregivers of my patients frequently ask me about the safety of their loved ones getting behind the wheel after receiving a diagnosis of AD. This is a sensitive topic for patients, but a very important one in terms of both safety and liability, as I will discuss here.

First, my own research has recently revealed that driving in moderate and late stage AD is a much larger problem than we first feared, and this is not attributable merely to aging. In fact, we have seen that 16-year-old males have a higher incidence of accidents than healthy non-demented individuals over the age of 75. However, in mild cognitive impairment (MCI) and the early stages of AD, we do not see increased accident rates. But as early AD progresses into moderate AD accident rates rise sharply.

Complicating things for the family is the fact that, according to state laws, the family could possibly be held liable if their loved one takes the car and gets into an accident. The family could be sued and held financially responsible.

As a physician, here are the things that I do with my patients, and suggest to others, to help support both the family and the patient, and especially to keep everyone involved safe and protected.

- The healthcare provider should assume responsibility – I always explain to my patients that I am a professional with a lot of experience in this area and based on their test results I believe that they should not be driving. I attempt to be very fact-based in this delivery, explaining the results of their test scores and indicate that they fall into a group with high accident rates.

- Next, I physically write a prescription and hand it to them, instructing them "no driving." This prescription goes home with them and is placed on the refrigerator, or bathroom mirror, or somewhere they will see it regularly.

- Sometimes I offer my patients a follow up call. This is a buffer to allow them time to adjust to the idea of not driving. In the office I tell them if they get home and still feel they need to discuss it, to give me a call back. I've made this offer over 500 times and no one has actually taken me up on it.

- I enable the family to agree with the patient, rather than argue. Family members can say "Hey, we agree with you about driving but, unfortunately the doctor said no, as you can see from this prescription. We cannot go against the doctor."

- If necessary, I encourage the family to disable the car – often after a couple of weeks the patient may simply stop inquiring about driving.

The best way to both support the patient and ease the stress on the family is for the healthcare provider to assume full responsibility for the decision to take away driving. If you are a caregiver with these concerns, talk to your healthcare provider privately and ask for support in making this decision.

Whatever you do, do not ignore the problem. This is a problem that can and does cost lives. If you doubt your loved ones ability to drive, do not allow it until you can receive further assessment from your physician. And above all, be sensitive in delivery of this news. Driving is a freedom that is very upsetting to part with and should not be taken lightly. Using these tips, the process should go much more smoothly for everyone involved.

CHAPTER 2

Dementia

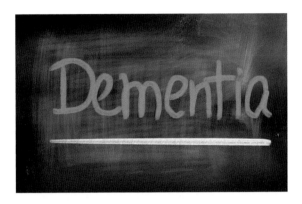

Dementia is a clinical syndrome characteristically marked by the gradual onset and slow progression of cognitive impairment. It involves a deficit in at least two cognitive domains and impairs one's ability to perform daily functions, i.e. job performance or social interactions. It must also be determined through testing that there is not another cause present, such as depression, vitamin deficiency or delirium. People often ask what is the difference between dementia and Alzheimer's disease (AD). The answer is that AD is a form of dementia.

There are several types of primary dementias:

Alzheimer's disease (AD) is the most common form of dementia and makes up around 60% of all cases. The most commonly affected domain in AD is memory. The progression of AD is slow, and it may be identifiable by some of these symptoms:

- Repeating questions (*attention* – the main domain affected)
- Trouble naming objects (*verbal fluency* – the second most common domain affected)
- Difficulty remembering appointments (*executive function*)
- Inability to balance a checkbook or handle financial transactions (*executive function*)
- Struggling to follow recipes when cooking (*executive function and memory*)

- Resistance to bathing and dressing; wearing the same clothing every day (*orientation*)
- Hoarding (*orientation*)

Many people with AD have difficulty with driving. One example is an individual who mistakenly got into the back seat of his car and began complaining because he thought someone had taken his steering wheel. This individual was very impaired but had no insight into his inability to operate an automobile. This individual has marked Anosognosia.

What is **Anosognosia**? Anosognosia is defined as "a real or feigned ignorance of the presence of a disease" according to Dr. Dougherty. Anosognosia is most commonly seen in patients with AD. This lack of ability to recognize one's disease is extremely important in AD, and especially important for family members to understand the problems with their loved one. About 50% of those with AD do not recognize that they have any problems and will admit no problems with memory when asked.

DEMENTIA

- Alzheimer's disease
- Dementia with Lewy bodies
- Vascular dementia
- Frontotemporal dementia
- Parkinson's related dementia

Dr. Dougherty describes some individuals with AD as being adept at having what he calls "cocktail party conversations" in that they can discuss the weather or talk about food even though they might not know what season it is outside. Problems arise when dealing with everyday situations. It is common for someone with AD to remember growing up or their first job but not remember what happened to them ten minutes ago.

If you have a loved one suffering with Anosognosia you are probably very familiar with this concept, even if you didn't know the medical term for it. AD patients with Anosognosia will argue with you if you point out deficits in memory or basic functioning. They tend to believe that they can function normally – still manage the finances, for example, when it is apparent to you that their cognitive deficits impair this ability.

AD patients with Anosognosia can be some of the toughest for caregivers to manage, and can create greater stress on loved ones. It may help to remember that this is a medical condition and that special care is needed to manage these individuals. It is often important to ensure that some individuals with Anosoagnosia do not drive, as this can present a dangerous situation.

It is frequently best not to argue with patients with Anosognosia when the issues are often of little consequence. Important issues however, should be dealt with firmly and directly, especially when it's time to explain to them that certain activities are dangerous for them, such as driving!

As the caregiver, always remember that patients with Anosognosia have a distorted self-awareness and are not just trying to be difficult.

Vascular dementia: This is the second most common cause of dementia in older adults, is usually preceded by many mini-strokes or TIAs (transient ischemic attacks) and is often detected by MRI scans. Patients who have vascular dementia typically exhibit more aggressive behavior. Vascular dementia tends to have a quicker onset. Suddenly, a person who was normally very calm may begin acting out. It is a shock to the system, and the individual then appears very confused.

The cognitive impairment associated with vascular dementia often is recognizable by early abnormalities of executive function. Visual-spatial abnormalities are common, as well. Memory is often mildly affected. There is frequently a significant abnormality of gait and occasionally, urinary incontinence may be present.

Diffuse Lewy body disease (DLB): This is a form of the primary dementias and makes up around 10-15% of all cases. Those with DLB often have visual hallucinations and can exhibit Parkinsonian traits—such as tremors, gait difficulties and falling. For example, I had one patient who was able to describe a hallucination in vivid detail of a purple rabbit with seven white whiskers. Another patient saw a garden gnome with red pants, a white hat, and nine fingers every time she looked out the window.

Fronto-temporal dementia (FTD): Among the major forms of dementia, FTD typically is a behavior variant where patients often say things that are inappropriate (known as behavioral dyscontrol). Frequently, there are striking abnormalities of executive function and problems with visual-spatial tasks. One example of a patient with FTD is someone who was usually quiet or reserved, but in a social situation such as going out to dinner, the patient might start talking to the people at a table nearby. As FTD progresses, the patient then might sit at the table next to theirs; and finally, he or she would sit at the table next to theirs and begin eating the food off their plates. FTD patients are aggressive in the way they talk, but the vast majority of them don't act on what they are saying.

Primary progressive aphasia (PPA): This is the second most common form of FTD. A person with PPA usually has significant problems with language capabilities. This type of dementia affects a person's ability to finish simple tasks. People who have PPA may lose most of their vocabulary, although there is very little cognitive abnormality present in the early stages. Later in the disease there are abnormalities in memory and executive function.

Progressive supranuclear palsy (PSP): This dementing illness is associated with striking problems with eye movements. There is often a significant abnormality of vertical gaze and the individual with PSP is known to have frequent falls. While the memory may remain intact, there are often significant abnormalities of executive function and visual-spatial abilities. For example, someone with PSP may be crying all the time; but it doesn't mean he or she is actually sad. It's all part of the disease.

Posterior cortical atrophy (PCA) – also called Benson's syndrome: This is a rare, degenerative neurological condition that often begins with visual complaints. These individuals do not struggle with acuity, but rather have problems with finding objects in space. Typical symptoms include difficulties with reading, and recognizing faces or common objects. Later in the disease, there are abnormalities of memory and verbal fluency.

Parkinson's related dementia. This form of dementia is associated with Parkinson's disease, presents differently than Alzheimer's disease and includes problems in executive function and visual spatial domains rather than a significant abnormality of memory.

SECONDARY DEMENTIAS

Secondary dementias, for the most part, begin with disease outside the nervous system. They are not associated with a degenerative process like Alzheimer's disease in which the pathology usually involves the brain itself and no other parts of the body. The secondary dementias usually involve some general systemic process that affects the brain secondarily. One important issue to remember about secondary dementias is that in many cases they are treatable dementias. These secondary dementias are divided into groups; infection, metabolic, brain tumors and trauma.

Infectious Disease

Cruetzfeldt-Jakob disease (CJD) - is sometimes referred to as mad-cow disease. CJD is a disease caused not by a virus but by an infectious protein very similar to a virus. In the past it was quite difficult to diagnosis CJD because there was not adequate neuro-imaging. In the past physicians would perform brain biopsies to diagnose CJD, but in association with this biopsy there was the potential for the spread of the disease itself. Now as one recent article suggests, MRI scans with contrast show abnormalities of the cortical ribbon in the frontal areas. These findings represent a typical picture associated with CJD and assist greatly in the diagnosis of this condition. Symptoms of CJD include rapid progression of memory loss, behavioral changes, poor coordination and visual-spatial problems. About 90% of individuals diagnosed with CJD die within one year.

AIDS dementia complex - is a dementia associated with HIV/AIDS and used to be more common. It's of particular interest because the brain is one of the few if not the only organ in the body that is actually invaded by the abnormal virus like particle associated with HIV/AIDS. AIDS dementia complex has undergone a dramatic change as it has become much less common with the new and helpful treatments for HIV/AIDS. "Twenty years ago I saw 5 patients a year with AIDS dementia complex and in 2013 I saw zero," Dr. Dougherty reports. Symptoms can include short attention span, memory problems, gait issues and behavioral changes.

Cryptococcal meningitis – this usually occurs in individuals who have immune suppression, for example, a patient with leukemia or AIDS. In the past it was difficult to diagnosis but we now have antigen antibodies that can identify it relatively easily, even from the peripheral blood. Symptoms include hallucinations, fever, nausea and vomiting and some mental changes. These symptoms can occur over days or weeks.

Metabolic states

Thyroid dysfunction - one of the most common metabolic states is thyroid disease, particularly hypothyroidism. "I saw an executive person recently who was complaining of difficulty with memory, unsteadiness, and weight gain. Examination showed that the individual was markedly hypothyroid and improved dramatically with treatment," said Dr. Dougherty. The positive treatment outcome associated with treating hypothyroidism reemphasizes the idea that many of these secondary dementias are indeed treatable.

Deficiency states

Vitamin B12 deficiency – the most common deficiency state is a vitamin B12 deficiency. B12 deficiency is an uncommon diagnosis but in my experience it almost always involves the peripheral nerves even prior to involving the brain. The name for B12 deficiency used to be "combined degeneration" and this is because it involved the brain, the nerves themselves, as well as a cognitive impairment. Symptoms include weakness, upset stomach and memory loss.

Toxins

The specific toxins discussed here are heavy metals and the abuse of alcohol and drugs. More specifically the heavy metals associated with cognitive changes consist of mercury, lead, cadmium and possibly arsenic. There are also reports of people having skin toxicity from mercury causing a multi symptom disease but also involving abnormalities of the brain and cognitive function. The continuous long-term abuse of alcohol and drugs has been shown to increase the possibility of cognitive impairment.

Some recent studies have shown that a relatively small amount of alcohol, this includes two glasses of wine for men and one glass for women, actually may have some preventative effect for AD.

Think of risk factors as "nature versus nurture" or "genetics versus environment and lifestyle".

Brain Tumors

Individuals may present with weakness and confusion associated with a brain tumor. "I saw one patient who was complaining of headaches and weakness. In retrospect the patient had some symptoms that made me suspect AD. After an appropriate examination it became clear he had lung cancer that had metastasized to the brain. This can happen, particularly in patients who have frontal lesions. When the lesion is more posterior one can have weakness in the arm or leg and the diagnosis is much more obvious. When the lesion is anterior the diagnosis may be much more difficult" explained Dr. Dougherty.

Trauma

A subdural hematoma (SDH) is a blood clot on the surface of the brain usually caused by trauma. Older adults with SDH frequently present with a new onset of headaches. It is very important to take that particular clinical syndrome, new onset headaches, and evaluate it carefully if they have not had a history of headaches.

Normal Pressure Hydrocephalus

Normal pressure hydrocephalus (NPH) - commonly referred to as "water on the brain" is associated with an increase in spinal fluid within the brain cavities. In the past the diagnosis of NPH was difficult because we did not have adequate tools to measure spinal fluid pressure over time. We now have new techniques which may identify the prognosis after inserting a shunt. A shunt is tubing that reduces brain spinal fluid pressure by draining the fluid into the abdominal cavity. This allows us to identify patients that would improve with a shunt thus improving the long-term outcomes of those with NPH.

CHAPTER 3

RISK FACTORS AND COGNITIVE SCREENING

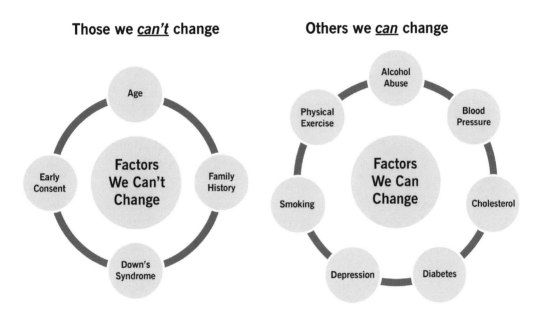

Those we _can't_ change

Age

Early Consent

Factors We Can't Change

Family History

Down's Syndrome

Others we _can_ change

Alcohol Abuse

Physical Exercise

Blood Pressure

Smoking

Factors We Can Change

Cholesterol

Depression

Diabetes

The risk factors for AD or other forms of dementia are divided into two categories: those that we **can** change and those we **cannot** change.

Risk factors we can't change

The number one risk factor for dementia is age. About one of every eight people has the chance of having AD by the time that individual is 65 years old. By the age of 85 there is a 45% chance of developing AD. Today, there are over 5.4 million people with AD in the United States, and 200,000 of those have early onset AD. Based purely on our aging population and the Baby Boomers reaching 65, the number of people with AD is expected to double every 20 years. These are somewhat staggering statistics, but remember that individuals will have to live to age 85 first!

AD is more common in females and there is an increased incidence of AD in those with a family history of the disease. The risk of AD for individuals with a family history is around 10%. But in many cases, people whose parents had or have early-onset dementia, typically before age 60, will have an increased chance of getting early onset AD.

Early-onset Alzheimer's disease occurs in people ranging in age from 30 to 60. It is rare, representing less than 3% of all individuals who have AD. In almost all cases, it is caused by genetic mutations of certain chromosomes and these mutations are inherited from a parent. Early-onset AD is also known as familial Alzheimer's disease (FAD). Several large-scale clinical trials have been launched over the past several years focused on populations known to possess the genetic mutations associated with FAD.

> Think of risk factors as "nature versus nurture" or "genetics versus environment and lifestyle".

Risk factors we can change

The good news is that there are several risk factors we can change by taking an active approach to our brain health.

Studies show a correlation between alcohol abuse and an increased chance of dementia. Generally, consuming more than 14 drinks per week can increase cell loss in the brain and cause atrophy.

Older individuals with high cholesterol and elevated blood pressure also tend to have a higher risk of AD. There is a direct correlation between keeping your heart healthy and decreasing your risk for AD. In addition, chronic smoking and tobacco use can lead to an increased propensity for AD, as can diabetes. Studies show that depression and high stress levels increase the potential for developing AD, and may also speed up its progression. Perhaps one of the most important factors in decreasing your chances for AD is physical exercise. Did you know that an increase in education level also has been shown to reduce the chance of getting AD?

Depression

Depression is a very important issue in regards to older adults. The rate of depression increases in older adults as does the rate of suicide. It is important to understand that there are very good and effective treatments for depression and many of these treatment options have relatively few side effects.

Depression can produce cognitive changes but the pattern is usually very different from AD in that it involves more pronounced attention abnormalities. In addition, symptoms of depression may increase cognitive abnormalities in patients with early AD.

It is said that approximately 20% of individuals who present with AD have an associated depression. This is a very important concept because patients that have a dementia or AD actually can have a substantial superimposed depression and therefore the effects can be synergistic. The depression may exacerbate the cognitive problem itself and treatment of depression can be very gratifying.

Apathy and delusions

Apathy has been largely underrated as a feature of AD, but it is not an uncommon symptom, especially in the later stages of the disease. An individual will spend hours sitting in a chair and watching TV, or lying in bed and being inactive much of the day.

Delusion can be associated with AD as well. Here Dr. Dougherty describes an individual with severe delusions. "Recently a patient had 2 sisters die within a month of each other, but she still felt they were alive, even though she had attended their funerals. The mechanism for storing historical information is not working properly so she was unable to focus on the idea that the sisters are, in fact, deceased."

Some individuals persistently believe a deceased spouse is still living and is still in the home with them. This type of delusion can be one of the emotional and behavioral manifestations of early AD as well.

METABOLIC SYNDROME

What is metabolic syndrome?

Metabolic syndrome is a collection of conditions that include increased blood pressure, high blood sugar levels, excess body fat around the waist or high cholesterol levels. When any of these risk factors occur together they increase your risk of heart disease, type 2 diabetes, stroke and dementia. If you have metabolic syndrome or any of the components of metabolic syndrome it is important to make certain lifestyle changes to delay or prevent serious health problems.

High Blood Pressure (Hypertension)

Blood pressure is a measure of how much force your blood puts against the arteries in your body. When the force of the blood against the arterial walls is too high it eventually causes health problems like heart disease, kidney disease and stroke. Your blood pressure measurement is determined 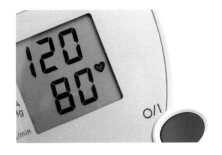 by the amount of blood your heart pumps and the amount of resistance to blood flow in your arteries. The more blood your heart pumps and the narrower your arteries, the higher your blood pressure. High blood pressure can develop slowly, so you can have high blood pressure for years without any symptoms but once you know you have high blood pressure you can work with your doctor to control it. Optimal blood pressure is defined as 120/80 – with a range of 120 – 129 / 80 – 89. Higher ranges are described as Grades of hypertension.

Blood Pressure	Range
Normal Range / Desired	120-80
High-normal Range	130 - 90
High-normal Range Age 60+	150 - 90
Grade 1 Hypertension	140 - 100
Grade 2 Hypertension	160 - 110
Grade 3 Hypertension or Hypertensive Crisis	>180 - >110

In early 2014 new hypertension recommendations indicate doctors should consider prescribing blood-pressure medications for patients age 60 and over whose levels are 150/90 or higher. The previous recommendation was 140/90. Your physician will determine your risks and prescribe medications accordingly.

High Blood Sugar – Diabetes

Diabetes is defined as a chronic disease in which an individual has high levels of sugar in their blood. Diabetes is caused either by too little insulin, resistance to insulin or both. People with diabetes have high blood sugar levels because the body is not able to store enough sugar for energy. There are two classifications of diabetes—Type 1 and Type 2. The latter type usually occurs in adults. One of the complications of diabetes is damage to the blood vessels. This affects all your major organs including the brain. Normal blood sugar levels have been established. Ideally, you want your fasting blood sugar level to be between 70 and 100. A major risk factor for becoming diabetic is being overweight.

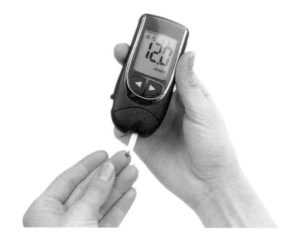

Blood Glucose Levels	Fasting (mg/dL)	2 nrs. Post Meal (mg/dL)
Normal	70 - 100	Less than 140
Early Diabetes	101 - 126	140 - 200
Diabetes	>126	>200

According to the American Diabetes Association's 2012 statistics, 29.1 million Americans, 9.3% of the population, have diabetes. It is estimated 86 million Americans age 20 and older have pre-diabetes.

High Cholesterol

High blood cholesterol is a major risk factor for heart disease and dementia. In fact the higher your blood cholesterol level the greater your risk for having a heart attack. Being "heart healthy" is directly related to being "brain healthy," so minimizing your risk for heart disease influences your risk for developing dementia.

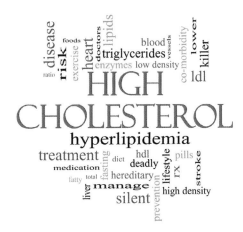

Cholesterol, often referred to as "plaque", is a fat-like substance in your blood that can build up along the walls of your arteries. When too much of this plaque builds up over time it causes "hardening of the arteries." This narrowing of your arteries affects the flow of blood and oxygen to vital organs, most importantly your heart and brain. High cholesterol does not cause symptoms so people may not be aware when their cholesterol levels are abnormal. It is important for your physician to check your cholesterol levels on a regular basis. Cholesterol levels are reported as total cholesterol, HDL and LDL. HDL is your "good" cholesterol and LDL is your "bad" cholesterol. You want your total cholesterol value to be under 200 and your HDL level to be as high as possible.

Cholesterol Level	Total Cholesterol
Desired	Less than 200
Borderline High	200 - 239
High Cholesterol	>240

The American Heart Association and American College of Cardiology released new cardiovascular prevention guidelines in late 2013. Physicians are encouraged to focus on lifestyle, cholesterol, obesity and risk assessment.

Subjective Cognitive Decline

A topic that has recently gained considerable interest and attention is the concept of subjective cognitive changes. That is to say individuals report that they have some difficulty in memory and perhaps other cognitive domains as well, but when tested their results using an objective cognitive test do not detect a cognitive abnormality.

The concept of subjective cognitive decline (SCD) becomes more difficult to ascertain when an individual has a negative cognitive assessment and a positive biomarker, e.g. a positive amyloid PET scan. It does appear that those with SCD and a positive amyloid scan have an increased rate of conversion to MCI or dementia.

There are many terms that have been used to categorize those individuals with early cognitive complaints. Some of these terms are "subjective memory impairment," "self-reported cognitive concerns," "subjective memory complaints" and "subjective cognitive concerns."

SCD is based on an individual's own feelings and not on objective cognitive tests. It is also important to understand it is not specifically associated with memory but includes the other cognitive domains including verbal fluency, executive function, visual-spatial, attention and orientation.

One study suggests that individuals who reported SCD have a 2.8 times greater risk of conversion to MCI or dementia. It is important to remember that although there is a greater risk for older adults who complain of cognitive difficulties, it does not mean that one will have a diagnosis of MCI or dementia.

Why is it important to screen for cognitive impairment?

A report commissioned by Alzheimer's Disease International titled "The Benefits of Early Diagnosis and Intervention," states that in high-income countries only 20% to 50% of dementia cases are recognized and documented in the primary care setting. In low and middle-income countries, this proportion could be as low as 10%. An estimated 90% of the people with mild cognitive impairment (MCI) go undiagnosed.

To study the prevalence of undiagnosed dementia and its related health care costs, the Minneapolis VA Medical Center gave a simple memory test to over 8,000 older adult primary care patients without a diagnosis of MCI. Over 25% of these patients failed the memory test and 95% of those who agreed to a formal neurological evaluation were diagnosed with cognitive impairment (76%

with dementia). This demonstrates an essential need for a sensitive cognitive screening tool in the primary care setting.

Benefits of Early Screening

Screening for the cognitive changes associated with cognitive impairment has become a major healthcare challenge. Most individuals who would benefit from cognitive screening are over the age of 65 and covered by Medicare.

Medicare has provided instructions to physicians to evaluate individuals for "cognitive changes" at the time of their Annual Wellness Visit (AWV) – an office visit focused on performing an overall health risk assessment and preparing a Personalized Prevention Plan based on the findings of that visit. Because this brief cognitive assessment is lumped in with the other evaluations, most physicians will ask their patients a few questions related to thinking and memory but do not perform specific cognitive tests during the AWV.

But a physician can assess you or a loved one for cognitive changes at any time. If you feel you need further evaluation or if you feel a loved one needs further evaluation because of concerns about memory, behavior or thinking abilities, please let your physician know and they will either conduct tests themselves or refer you to a neurologist for a complete neurologic evaluation.

A recent report on cognitive screening from the U.S. Preventive Services Task Force indicates up to 81% of individuals who meet the criteria for dementia have never received a documented diagnosis.

A delay in making a diagnosis or missing a diagnosis deprives individuals of being able to seek available treatments and create care plans with healthcare, legal and caregiver professionals. Many may miss an opportunity to use community support services. It is important to remember that primary and secondary caregivers benefit from an early and accurate diagnosis as well. It gives everyone time to plan for the future while the individual is still able to participate in the decision making processes.

Treatments for Alzheimer's disease and other dementias have been minimally effective in clinical trials mainly because the conditions are not caught early enough. A recent survey published in Alzheimer's Research and Therapy indicates interest in early medical testing for Alzheimer's disease is high. Individuals with high levels of perceived risk – those who worried about getting AD because they are a caregiver or have a blood relative with AD – are among those most likely to pursue testing.

Benefits of Early Screening:
- Increased understanding of the different types of dementia

- Make lifestyle adjustments to promote healthy living (exercise, diet, minimize stress)
- Start medications
- Explore participating in a clinical trial to help advance research
- Plan for the future by participating in decisions about care, transportation, living options, financial and legal matters
- Develop a relationship with your doctors and care partners
- Use and benefit from community support services
  and
- Allay concerns if all the tests are negative.

How we can help!

The COGselftest is a reliable screening tool that can help in the early identification of cognitive impairment, AD or other form of dementia. By using the COGselftest, medical professionals and consumers will begin to recognize that they can do something to help monitor and protect cognitive function. Together, we will change the perception of Alzheimer's disease.

▾ Comparison of **cog**selftest and MMSE diagnostic accuracy rates

| 95% ACCURACY | **cog**selftest |
| 67% ACCURACY | MMSE |

▾ Comparison of **cog**selftest and MMSE in detecting cognitive impairment

| 97% NORMAL VS. AD | **cog**selftest |
| 83% NORMAL VS. AD | MMSE |

The MMSE (Mini-Mental State Exam) is a widely used, validated, and reliable method of screening for Alzheimer's disease.

The information provided by COGselftest empowers consumers to be proactive about their brain health. Knowing areas of cognitive deficiencies will help individuals and their caregivers choose appropriate ways to preserve and protect cognitive, mental and physical health.

The COGselftest allows for easy and reliable early screening, leading to peace of mind. This suggests that AD or another type of dementia can be identified in its earliest stages when interventions are most effective.

Screening in the Public Environment

The COGselftest™ is also available directly to the public on-line. Individuals can take the COGselftest in less than 10 minutes, test all 6 cognitive domains, download, save and print a report they can share with their personal care physician at any time. The test results also provide domain specific tasks focused on strengthening each domain and improving overall brain health. This is the same test given in the physician office setting.

Understanding your COGselftest results

The results and a personalized prevention plan are automatically generated after the completion of the COGselftest. These results are saved to your account and can be printed, saved or emailed. They are broken down by each cognitive domain:

Visual Spatial

Executive Function

Verbal Fluency

Memory

Attention

Orientation

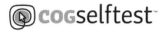

Results of your **COG**selftest™

Your COGselftest Results for **December 31st, 2014** 9:33am EDT.

Your results indicate early warning markers in Orientation, Attention, Verbal Fluency, Memory, Visual Spatial, and Executive Functions. Since you missed questions in multiple cognitive domains, it is recommended that you print your results and take them to your physician for further evaluation. Your physician will be able to access our site for further details and information about your test (with your permission). Again, this is an early warning screening test, not a diagnosis. Only your physician can make a diagnosis. But we can help educate you and family members about scientifically proven ways to delay symptoms of cognitive impairment. That's why we are here.

Recent studies have shown there are many ways to keep our brains stimulated and our mental function optimal. Once you have reviewed your results below, click on each domain to learn more and print out the exercises to keep your mental function and peak performance. And be sure to sign up for our newsletter to stay up to date on the latest news and research on Alzheimer's Disease.

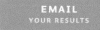 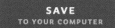 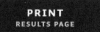

SEE HOW YOU RANK AMONG YOUR PEERS ▶

YOUR RESULTS BY COGNITIVE DOMAIN

1. Visual Spatial   BELOW AVERAGE

You need to improve your Visual Spatial.
A visual spatial defect means that you have difficulty localizing objects in a two or three dimensional space. For example you might have difficulty ...**READ MORE**

   IMPROVE YOUR SKILLS WITH THESE EXERCISES

2. Executive Functions   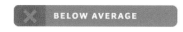 BELOW AVERAGE

You need to improve your Executive Function.
he executive system is a theorized function of psychology that controls and manages other cognitive processes. The concept is used by psychologists and neuroscientists ...**READ MORE**

   IMPROVE YOUR SKILLS WITH THESE EXERCISES

3. Verbal Fluency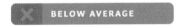

You need to improve your Verbal Fluency.
As defined, Verbal Fluency is the ability to create language. Have you ever tried to think of a word and it is at the tip of the tongue but you can't come up with it? ...**READ MORE**

   IMPROVE YOUR SKILLS WITH THESE EXERCISES

4. Memory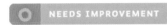

You have room to improve in your Memory.
>Memory is the ability to recall events that happened in the past. We examine memory by giving a person a number of words to remember then giving them a distraction ...**READ MORE**

   IMPROVE YOUR SKILLS WITH THESE EXERCISES

5. Attention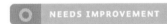

You have room to improve in your Attention.
Attention is the cognitive process of selectively concentrating on one aspect of the environment while ignoring other things. Attention has also been referred to ...**READ MORE**

   IMPROVE YOUR SKILLS WITH THESE EXERCISES

6. Orientation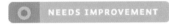

You have room to improve in your Orientation.
Orientation is simply your awareness of yourself in time, place, and location. We examine one's orientation abilities by seeing asking the day, month, year and by going ...**READ MORE**

   IMPROVE YOUR SKILLS WITH THESE EXERCISES

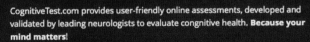

ABOUT   YOUR BRAIN   COGSELFTEST   TESTIMONIALS   FAQ   CONTACT US

CognitiveTest.com provides user-friendly online assessments, developed and validated by leading neurologists to evaluate congnitive health. **Because your mind matters!**

Delay the onset!

Alzheimer's disease usually develops slowly, so it can be many years before symptoms are noticeable. Early screening can highlight symptoms long before they become disabling.

If the onset of AD could be delayed for five years, it would effectively reduce the number of patients with the disease by half because it is such a late life disease.

The COGselftest is a screening tool for cognitive impairment and does not provide a diagnosis of AD. Unlike existing tests for cognitive impairment, the COGselftest looks at each cognitive domain separately. The test results provide a detailed description of each cognitive domain. Your performance in each domain is then compared to age matched controls.

Your test results are divided into three (3) categories for each cognitive domain: Excellent, Needs Improvement and Below Average. This allows you to work on specific areas that may slow the progression of any cognitive problems. Clicking on each domain provides you with specific tasks you can do to improve in those areas. It is important that you continue to test yourself over time so that you can determine changes in your cognitive function as you age. The more you use your brain, the better chance you have for neuronal stimulation and rehabilitation. Use it or lose it!

CHAPTER 4

Your Six Cognitive Domains

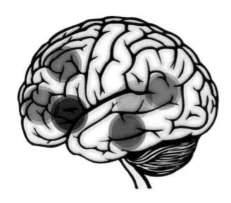

Did you know that any activity you do is controlled by your "cognitive domains" and that there are six of them? When figuring out how to enhance and protect your cognitive health, the first step is to understand these six areas of the brain. "Cognition" deals with the set of skills or processes used to comprehend and interact with the world. Your cognitive abilities have to do with how you learn, recall, problem-solve and manifest attention. For example, answering the phone involves hearing the ring tone and reacting (perception and decision-making, motor-skills and language abilities). It also includes social skills (responding to another voice).

Scientists are researching ways to help prevent or stall cognitive decline, as seen in Alzheimer's disease and other types of dementia.

The COGselftest is the only early-warning online screening test that measures the six cognitive domains.

VISUAL SPATIAL

A "visual spatial" weakness means that you may have difficulty focusing on objects in a two-or-three dimensional space. For example, you might have trouble setting the table, putting blocks together, or even drawing a clock.

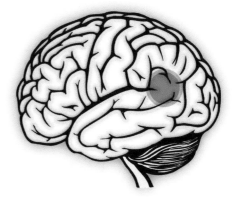

Individuals with visual-spatial deficits are prone to getting lost because they cannot visualize how to get back.

An extreme example often observed in people with visual spatial issues is in locating and identifying specific objects, such as pointing to the doorknob in a room. The person will not be able to recognize specific parts on the door—and instead sees the whole door or the wall. But when that person is asked to leave the room, he or she will walk straight to the doorknob and open the door.

Changes in the occipital lobe and associated areas of the parietal and temporal lobes are the usual causes of these deficits. Ask someone to describe how he or she gets from a room to the kitchen. A person with a visual spatial deficit will have trouble formalizing a map in his or her head and then describing the layout.

"I have a patient whose family was concerned because their family member was not able to wrap a present. She was able to put the bow on top of the package but was not able to measure and cut the appropriate amount of wrapping paper to cover the box. This is an example of someone with a visual-spatial deficit."
– Dr. Dougherty

EXECUTIVE FUNCTION

Can you tell me how bicycles and cars are alike? Or, what do a clock and a watch have in common? The answer is "transportation" and both the clock and the watch tell time. But for someone with issues in "executive function," he or she might not be able to come up with these answers.

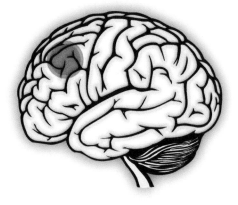

In general terms, think of your executive function as being able to do abstract thinking. The executive system concept is used by psychologists and neuroscientists to describe a collection of brain processes, which are responsible for:

• Planning and cognitive flexibility
• Abstract thinking
• Rule acquisition

• Initiating appropriate actions and inhibiting inappropriate actions
• Selecting relevant sensory information

A way to test executive function is to ask what a common saying means. For example, describe what this phrase means to you: "People in glass houses shouldn't throw stones." A normal response might be as follows: "People shouldn't criticize the faults of others when they have faults themselves." Often someone with executive function problems might be too literal and tell you that if you throw stones you will break the glass house—instead of being able to think abstractly. Executive function issues are often linked with ADHD (Attention Deficit Hyperactivity Disorder).

Individuals diagnosed with fronto-temporal dementia (FTD) will often have severe executive function issues, for example, someone with FTD will act out or become socially disinhibited.

VERBAL FLUENCY

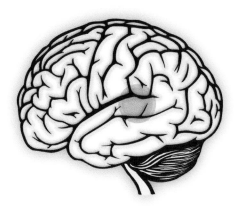

Verbal fluency is defined as the ability to generate language. The level of verbal fluency includes how rapidly you can come up with language or how quickly your brain accesses your vocabulary. Whether you are having a quick, witty conversation or trying to come up with an author of your favorite book, your degree of verbal fluency is often affected with aging. The good news is that it often helps for a person with verbal fluency problems to play word-association games.

Have you ever tried to think of a word and it's on the tip of your tongue but you can't come up with it? An example often seen is when someone is trying to come up with the word "clock." He or she will be able to say it has hands and numbers, but the word "clock" cannot be recalled.

Verbal fluency is the second most common domain affected in Alzheimer's disease and is not tested in several of the more common cognitive screenings.

MEMORY

"Memory" is the ability to recall events that happened in the past. We examine memory by giving a person a number of words to remember, and then assigning a "distraction task" that can last from 2-5 minutes. Next, we ask the person to recall those words. This tests the ability in short-term memory retention.

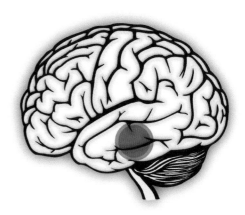

A memory decline is usually the first symptom of cognitive impairment. And, the number one risk factor for memory loss is age. Memory is also the most common deficit associated with Alzheimer's disease, and often is what frightens people the most about aging. We often see people start or end the test by telling stories about when they were younger. For example, we tested one individual who did not perform well, but after the test he went into vivid detail about his career in the army. Family members or even the person with memory loss will believe there is no issue because they can recall in detail events that happened to them in the past. Simply put, being able to remember events that happened 20 years ago does not mean there are no memory problems.

There is a difference between working memory and short-term memory. Working memory consists of keeping information current in your mind for a short timeframe in order to use it for the task you are dealing with at the moment. It is supported by the frontal regions and the parietal areas of the brain. Working memory uses short-term memories for effecting behaviors. For example, if you walk into an office, the direction you turn at each hall is in your short-term memory. The processing of that information such that one can backtrack and find your way out of the office involves working memory. It involves the executive and attention aspects of short-term memory in that you are able to integrate, process and retrieve information.

Another form of memory is motor memory – otherwise known as your muscle memory. The most common example of motor memory is "riding a bicycle" – in other words once the memory is learned and the function is repeated then it is committed to muscle memory. In AD muscle memory is often the last form of memory affected.

So, it's important to figure out how you can use this knowledge of how memory works to improve it. The first thing we tell someone who is seeking to bolster their memory is that they must first commit to improvement. If you are convinced there is nothing that can be done about your "bad" memory, then you will never improve.

ATTENTION

"Attention" is the cognitive process of selectively concentrating on one aspect of the environment while ignoring other things. It has also been referred to as the allocation of processing resources. Now what does this mean for a person suffering from cognitive impairment? Our experience shows that attention issues often show up in later-stage cognitive impairment or Alzheimer's disease.

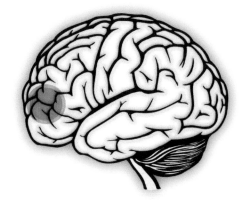

We might test attention by asking someone to name the months backwards. Another more difficult attention test is called the Serial Seven – where one is asked to subtract 7 from 100 five times. You might ask someone to follow a sequence that you provide. For example, "Every time I tap my leg, I want you to tap your shoulder; but if I tap my shoulder, I want you to tap your leg." This might seem basic or easy for you, but a person with attention problems will have trouble focusing enough to follow your lead.

I always ask my patients to "walk fancy" for me because their gait is not affected with Alzheimer's disease until the later stages. Gait is affected with other primary degenerative dementias like Parkinsonian dementia.

– Dr. Dougherty

You can improve your attention by keeping a regular sleeping schedule and working on your ability to focus attention. A study of healthy elderly subjects suggests that focused attention training can actually improve overall cognitive performance. I would recommend not only listening to a performance or watching a movie, but then have an open discussion about what happened in the movie or how the performance made the viewer feel.

ORIENTATION

Your "orientation" is simply the awareness of yourself in time, place, and location. Neurologists typically examine someone's orientation abilities by asking the day, month, and year. Then they will go more in-depth by asking that person where he or she is. For example, if a person is at a hospital, then we might ask what floor he or she is on. When we ask some older adults what the day or month is, we find that they might get flustered or give the incorrect

answer—even if they have no orientation
deficits. We often get the response, "I am
retired and I don't need to know what
the day is." Well, that is true to a certain
extent, but a lack of overall awareness
will only decrease one's overall cognitive
performance. If you are unaware of your
surroundings or simply don't care to know
the date, then you are in essence opening
yourself up to further problems in memory,
executive function, and general mental
wellbeing.

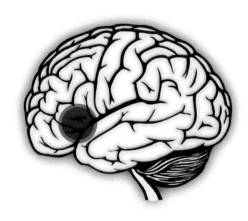

Early orientation problems often lead to depression, which can decrease
cognitive performance even further, as discussed in the previous section.
A solution is to keep older adults aware of their surroundings, engaged in
everyday activities,and make sure they see the value of being aware of oneself. A
simple way to help improve awareness within someone's home is to add a small
"white board" in a common area and write dates, activities, or other messages
on it. Another example that an Assisted Living Facility used was adopting a local
minor league baseball team. The residents were able to keep up with each game,
cheer for the team, and follow the progression of the season. Often, the players
would visit the facility or the residents would attend a game so that they were
personally involved with the team. This helped not only with orientation, but
also with overall cognitive performance and mood.

Which domains need attention?

Most people mistakenly believe that their cognitive well-being is only about
their memory. They think their memory is similar to the recording made by a
video camera. In fact, most people think that their brains can store records of
every experience in their lives.

But this is actually quite far from the truth. Typically, your brain cannot recall
something until it believes that the event or circumstance has had a significant
impact on your personal life. It truly demands that you are actively involved in
an experience in order to remember it.

Your brain has a surprising ability to forget things. It turns out that
throughout your entire life, your brain has done an excellent job at forgetting.
For example, can you remember your best friend's phone number from grade
school? There are so many inputs into our brain each day that we categorize
them by importance and how often we retrieve that input.

How will you know which is "natural forgetting" and which areas of your brain need more attention to prevent or delay dementia? An objective evaluation of your memory is often essential and the COGselftest is very useful in this regard.

Methods to improve each domain

We realize that it typically becomes more difficult to learn new things as people age. That's because the brain's processing speed is slowing down. It also is harder for the brain to multitask, and so it's easier to get confused. In addition, the aging brain is getting more set in its ways—so it is often more difficult to change the way the brain learns.

Researchers have not yet found a way to "upgrade your brain's hard drive" in the same way that a computer's hard drive is upgraded. However, there are many techniques to improve your brain's overall performance.

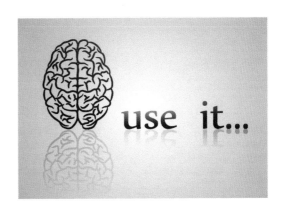

- Stay active
- Challenge yourself daily
- Learn new activities
- Remain independent
- Exercise

Suggested tasks for each Cognitive Domain

Visual Spatial

1. Practice copying forms, such as a 3-D box.
2. Create drawings and/or paintings of houses with skylines and gardens.
3. Practice drawing a clock with the numbers indicating the times you take your medications.
4. Practice tying complicated knots.
5. Purchase maze or puzzle books – note you can also find these online.
6. Practice writing down directions to the grocery store, church, etc.
7. Practice making origami figures.
8. Draw pictures with your grandchildren.
9. Play a game of Tetris.
10. Visit museums and observe how different artists arrange objects in space.

Executive Function

1. Learn a new activity like digital photography and learn to share pictures online.

2. Develop a financial plan, and keep track of your finances.
3. Organize plans for your yard work.
4. Host an event for family and/or friends.
5. Practice following recipes.
6. Follow the stock market.
7. Play What-if games or 20 Question games.
8. Organize your closet according to season.
9. Try playing games on-line; one example is play "A Google a Day"; http://www.agoogleaday.com/
10. Play cards with your family or friends or play solitaire on the Internet.

Verbal Fluency

1. Practice naming parts of the body.
2. Name objects in your living room.
3. Think of types of cars as you drive and practice naming them.
4. Think about ancestors and draw a family tree.
5. Work on following commands from an instruction book.
6. Learn how to do a new project; work on the computer.
7. Work on remembering names of people you meet.
8. Use word association to help you remember items.
9. Watch a movie then recall and discuss your favorite scenes.
10. Read books, this includes using electronic readers.

Memory

1. Keep track of your own medication schedule.
2. Play with flash cards.
3. Practice the names of friends, acquaintances or resent movie characters.
4. Practice balancing exercises to train muscle memory.
5. Sign up with brain training sites like Posit Science or Lumosity.
6. Learn and play "n-back" challenging type games.
7. Use a white board to document activities (make a time line).
8. Write down financial transactions in a checkbook or spreadsheet and keep notes.
9. Keep a journal for posterity.
10. Always place your keys and glasses in the same place.

Attention

1. Work on finishing a task to completion.
2. Try the Pomodoro Technique – a time management technique that uses a timer to break down your work schedule.

3. Meditate.
4. Join a book club.
5. Practice staying on subject during a conversation.
6. Spell words backward.
7. Set up and complete jigsaw puzzles.
8. Try new hobbies that keep you curious and engaged, like bird watching.
9. Remain focused on a single conversation in social situations.
10. Practice simple mathematics.

Orientation
1. Keep a calendar and an activity book.
2. Review your calendar on a daily basis.
3. Try and recall important events in history.
4. Read the newspaper and news magazines.
5. Check the Internet daily for current news or watch a newscast daily.
6. Follow a sports team and keep up with the game stats.
7. When you go on vacation, keep a careful record of where you are each day.
8. Keep a notepad that starts with today's date.
9. Track the birthdays and special events of friends and close family members.
10. Check the time of day at least every 2 hours.

Various other tasks to improve overall cognitive health:
- Ask about your medications, keep track of them and find out what they are needed for.
- Talk to family members and be honest about your worries and feelings.
- Be socially active.
- If you need answers to concerns regarding your health or relationships, consider seeing a counselor.
- Join social organizations.
- Set reachable goals for each day, week, and month.
- Practice following recipes, making multiple dishes and make sure they come out on time.
- Create lists ("to do" lists or shopping lists); check off each completed task or purchase.
- Take a class at a local university or community college.
- Eat regular scheduled meals, and try not to eat after 8 p.m.
- Go to bed at regular hours.
- Keep a sleep chart and a dream book; calculate the hours you sleep each day.

- Keep track of your bills, practice equations.
- Exercise – Yoga, Tai Chi, stretching; make sure to walk and do other forms of exercise at least 30 minutes most days each week.

Neuroscientists at the University of Texas at Dallas conducted a study with older adults to see if there was a difference in learning complex tasks and compared the outcome to a group performing less challenging tasks. Individuals who learned digital photography and Photoshop in addition to individuals who learned quilting showed the greatest improvement in memory. And this improvement lasted into the 1st year of testing. Challenging activities can strengthen entire networks in our brains, not just memory!

Sources

(Sybille Rockstroh)

(http://sharpbrains.com/blog/2010/11/16/what-is-working-memory-can-it-be-trained/)

(http://www.scientificamerican.com/article/experts-short-term-memory-to-long-term/)

(http://www.brainwaves.com/memory_concentration.html)

(https://www.youtube.com/watch?v=5rIf5pllw3U&feature=youtu.be)

(http://www.alz.org/professionals_and_researchers_13532.asp)

(http://sharpbrains.com/blog/2006/12/18/what-are-cognitive-abilities/)

(Gary Small, 2003)

CHAPTER 5

Body and Brain Fitness

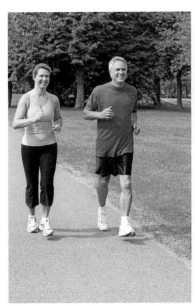
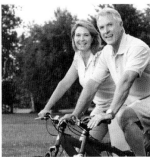
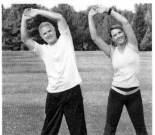

A study calculated that an intervention that would delay the onset of AD by 12 months would lead to 9.2 million fewer cases of AD globally. Research has estimated that reducing inactivity by 10-25% could prevent between 380,000 to one million cases of AD worldwide. Based on published reports, if the cost of care for an AD patient is $10,000 more per year than a patient without AD, we would save 3.8 to 10 billion dollars a year.

Despite the benefits of exercise, research suggests that the subpopulation of older adults actually exercise less. In general, health-promoting behaviors tend to increase with age, with the exception of exercise. Different factors as to why this age group is more sedentary include: lack of self-efficacy, inadequate education, poor support, limited access to recommended exercise and abnormalities of mobility. Isolation, cost, lack of socialization as well as poor physician emphasis are also factors.

Exercise is a cost effective, non-pharmaceutical treatment to delaying the onset of dementia and improves outcomes. A critical challenge is how to help older adults overcome obstacles that prevent them from developing a healthy exercise habit. One major obstacle is a lack of motivation for exercise.

A growing amount of research reveals that an "enriched" environment may be crucial to improving brain health. "Enriched" simply means that influences such as physical exercise and intellectual stimulation can affect your brain's functioning.

Findings from brain health studies at UC Berkeley have corroborated the importance of exercise on brain health. It all makes perfect sense, as the brain is a vital part of the body. Since it is comprised of cells nourished by your blood, your heart's health also plays an important role in your brain's wellbeing. Regular physical activity improves cerebral blood flow, which promotes better mental functioning. So, it's easy to see why both physical and intellectual exercises would help improve brain functioning.

> The important part is to find an exercise routine that fits your lifestyle. Studies show that it takes 28 days for an exercise routine to become a habit. Post your exercise schedule on your wall and set goals for yourself that you can accomplish each week.

Further, physical exercise also helps to lower stress—which is like a toxin to the brain. When cortisol, "the toxic stress hormone," is produced by the body as a result of stress, it lowers the glucose energy supply to the brain. This can create confusion and short-term memory issues. It can also affect the brain's chemicals that send messages from one cell to another. These chemicals are called neurotransmitters. If the stress is ongoing or chronic, the cortisol levels might get so high that it could be enough to kill brain cells and affect the development of Alzheimer's disease. Physical exercise and intellectual challenges can help to lower these cortisol levels. One recent study at Columbia University, suggests that exercise may even produce neurogenesis, the development of new neurons, in the hippocampus of the brain. Therefore, cardiovascular fitness is not the only advantage of exercise.

A study published in the Archives of Internal Medicine reports that individuals who start exercising in their 70s or 80s can prolong their lives

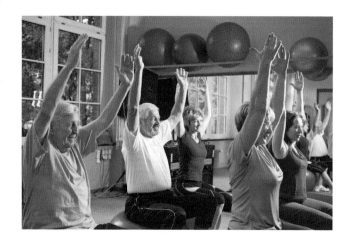

up to four years, and experience a lower risk of disability, compared to those who are sedentary. This is the first study to track those who begin exercising very late in life.

We have provided an exercise program and schedule for individuals with limited mobility.

Proposed Weekly Schedule for individuals with mobility restrictions

Many individuals may have mobility restrictions, so incorporating a routine exercise program can be challenging. If you already have a routine exercise program you follow, please keep it up. If not, we have provided a proposed weekly exercise schedule that can be modified based on your ability to move about. Many exercises we suggest are designed to be performed in a chair. We recommend you try to incorporate as many of these in your exercise plan as you can. Try to exercise 5 times a week.

Flexibility – *need a chair*

Balance – *need a chair and access to a step or stair or an exercise step device*

Strength – *may use 1 or 2 pound hand weights easy to grasp and hold on to*

Aerobic workout – *need a chair – preferably with arms*

Hand dexterity – *need a chair and a small ball that bounces (at least 8 inches in diameter)*

Monday Flexibility Exercises	Tuesday Balance	Wednesday Strength	Thursday Aerobic Workout	Friday Hand Dexterity
1. Sit on the floor and try to reach your toes. Do this one leg at a time, and then do both legs at the same time. Do 10 reps	1. While standing, lift yourself up on the toes of your feet and then relax back down on your flat feet. Do 10 reps	1. Consider using small 1 or 2 pound weights that are easy to grasp and hold on to and curl your bicep up to your shoulder. Do 10 reps with each arm	1. Sit in a chair with your feet flat on the ground and practice getting up and sitting back down. Alternate using your hands for support and trying to do it without using your hands. Do this 10 times	1. While seated, extend the fingers of one hand then close those fingers into a fist. Do 15 reps with each hand
2. While seated, put your hands behind your head and then slowly turn to the right and hold the position for 5 seconds. Alternate between your right & left. Do 5 reps each side	2. Using a step or stair or an exercise step product, step up and then step back down. Do 10 reps while alternating your starting foot	2. Standing or sitting, extend your arms outward (like you are punching) and bring each arm back one at a time. Do 20 reps alternating arms	2. While sitting in the chair, flat footed, lift one leg up in an extended form to your waist level and then lower it back to the floor. Do 10 reps with each leg	2. Clasp your hands together and extend and rotate your arms in a circular motion. Alternate between small circles and larger circles. Do 10 reps and then reverse the circles
3. Sitting or standing, cross your arms and put your hands in a fist. Open your hands and bring your arms up in the air with thumbs extended to make the shape of a "V" with your arms. Then make a fist again and bring your arms back to the original position. Do 10 reps – relaxing for a few seconds between each one	3. While standing, hold on to the back of a chair placed at your right side and raise your left leg up (bending the knee) and then straighten your left leg, hold it for 10 seconds, and place it back on the floor. Do 5 reps and then turn around in the other direction and hold the chair back with your left hand and do the exercise with your right leg. Do 5 reps	3. Lift your arms from your side to a full extension of your arm and hold for about 10 seconds. Do 10 reps with each arm or you can do this with both arms at the same time	3. When you can, take a 15 to 30-minute walk. Do this at least 5 times per week – or as often as possible. For some individuals it might be easier to "walk in place" for as long as you can – but at lease 15 minutes. You can walk in place while watching a favorite TV program!	3. Using a small ball, bounce it on the floor and then catch it, then throw it in the air overhead and catch it. Do 15 reps

More notes:
- Try to increase the repetitions for each exercise over time
- Make a chart and calendar and have participants keep up with their progress. This will help with overall orientation.
- When counting the repetitions for each exercise alternate counting forward and backwards.

Mental training for a better brain

Did you know that developing new skills actually spurs the growth of brand-new brain cells? When you take on new learning challenges, your neurons get fired up and you can literally build new connections between brain cells. You've probably already heard that doing crosswords can help improve your brain functioning. But if you do daily crosswords routinely, then it's really not enough. You truly need to change your routine to include other games such as bridge or Sudoku.

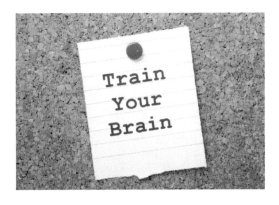

A preliminary study of older adults aged 65 to 91 who joined Facebook, friended others and posted at least once a day showed a 25% improvement in working memory.

Learning something new and novel provides the most benefit. Try learning the basics of a new language. Spend time on your computer visiting new sites that interest you. Do you like poetry? Visit your favorite poet's website or find poems online and read them aloud to yourself or a friend.

Some simple things like brushing your teeth with your non-dominant hand or combing your hair using the other hand can stimulate new neural connections. If you are an avid reader, change genres to stimulate your brain. If you like mysteries switch and read biographies for a while.

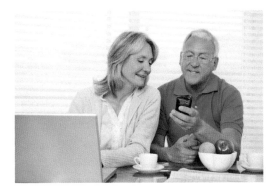

Recently, UCLA researchers using fMRI scanning discovered that older people could activate brain areas that involve complex reasoning and decision-making—after only one week of learning new

Internet skills. This demonstrates how learning new things can have a huge impact on preserving your brain functioning as you age.

What research has revealed about the brain

Here are a few "fun facts" that might motivate you to put on your thinking cap for the good of your brain:

- Each beat of your heart circulates one-quarter of the oxygen and blood to your brain.
- Everybody's brain has both a cortex and a sub-cortex.
- For most people, the brain's left hemisphere controls language.
- The right hemisphere of the brain is used for functions other than language (for most of the population).
- There is a hippocampus in each hemisphere of your brain, and each one can take in new information to spark learning.
- Each person has almost 100 billion neurons (brain cells) that can multiply as the person comes across new situations.
- Your brain cells send messages to one another in a connection called a "synapse."
- As your brain makes more connections, its reserve grows.
- This "brain reserve" is believed to hold off the onset of dementia.

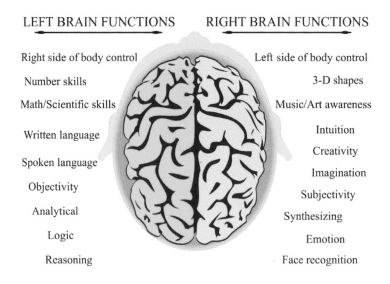

LEFT BRAIN FUNCTIONS	RIGHT BRAIN FUNCTIONS
Right side of body control	Left side of body control
Number skills	3-D shapes
Math/Scientific skills	Music/Art awareness
Written language	Intuition
Spoken language	Creativity
Objectivity	Imagination
Analytical	Subjectivity
Logic	Synthesizing
Reasoning	Emotion
	Face recognition

An important takeaway from this factoid list is that the brain is constantly changing throughout life's course. This is known as "brain plasticity" " or "neuro-plasticity," which really means that there's no limitation to the brain's capabilities. Of course, each person's gray matter is unique and truly superior to the most powerful computer.

Over a lifetime—starting at birth—everyone's brain is affected by the input received from the environment. The type of input will definitely influence the health of your brain. So that's why it's so important to make that input count!

You have some control over the kind of messages your brain receives. By taking charge, you can promote your own brain's well-being.

Sources:
(http://www.aarp.org/health/brain-health/info-01-2012/boost-brain-health.html)
(http://www.leadered.com/pdf/Build_Brain_Healthy_Environment_2014.pdf)
(http://sharpbrains.com/blog/2006/08/13/physical-fitness-and-brain-fitness/)

CHAPTER 6

Nutrition for a Healthier Brain

Before you sit down to your next plate of pasta, veggies or broiled fish, have you ever considered whether these foods are good for your body and brain? Most people only think about keeping their body fit on the outside, and forget about their brain health. Did you know that your brain is involved in nearly everything you do— from sleeping to walking to reading? So keeping your gray matter healthy is vital for your overall well-being.

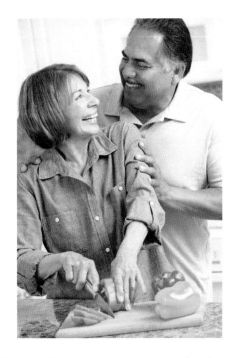

Here's food for thought: Research has confirmed that as people age, their poor nutritional habits would place them at a higher risk for several health-related problems, including: heart disease, type 2 diabetes, high cholesterol, high blood pressure, strokes, osteoporosis and some forms of cancer. As a general rule, findings also show that good nutrition for the body is good for the brain.

Nutrition and brain health

For more than 18 years I have worked with medical teams at the University of Tennessee to follow over 3,000 patients with Alzheimer's disease (AD). As neurologists, we were slow to realize how diet could affect brain health. We know that diabetes, high blood pressure, and heart disease increase the risk for AD. However, recent studies show how nutrition can affect the aging process. It turns out that particular nutrients and chemicals are important for proper brain function and that people who don't "feed the brain" with foods that contain them may impair their cognitive function. (Note: "Cognition" is the ability to take information and use it to deal with daily life matters.)

It is essential that our aging population preserve their brains, especially because their life quality, independence and economic status may depend on it. If you are among this population, it's urgent that you understand how your brain is handling information with each passing year. You might be able to make a change for the better by watching what you eat. Therefore, it is imperative to generate a nutritional plan that focuses on optimizing your energy intake. By doing so, you will get a jump-start on protecting your brain cells.

Protecting your brain cells

Put your worries aside and begin feeding your brain the foods that research has found will help protect it. Guarding your brain's health starts with impacting its neurotransmitters. These are chemicals released from a nerve cell, which then transmit an impulse to another nerve, muscle, organ or tissue. Known as the "messengers" between brain cells, neurotransmitters serve as communication pathways for information to flow from one cell to another.

The good news is that some neurotransmitters can be directly impacted through the diet:

Serotonin	Dopamine	Norepinephrine	Acetylcholine
• Mood • Anxiety • Sleep • Sensitivity	• Movement • Attention • Learning • Mood • Pleasure	• Concentration • Alertness	• Voluntary muscle movement • Behavior inhibition • Memory

DHA and EPA are orthomolecules whose functional sites are exclusively cell membranes, where they interact with other fatty acids to maintain fluidity. They are found in highest concentrations in the most dynamic membranes (i.e., the brain, retina, and spermatozoa). Scientific literature on DNA confirms that it is essential for normal neurological development, maintenance of learning and memory, and brain plasticity.

– Wu, Ying, and Gomez Pinilla; research study

Your everyday eating habits

Here are some ways to ramp up the "healthy" in your daily nutrition routine:

- √ Eat regularly scheduled meals
- √ Avoid food without nutritional value (most processed foods)
- √ Regulate your caloric intake
- √ Include a variety of food groups in your diet

Diets with omega-3 fatty acids

A most common recommendation for your diet is to increase the intake of omega-3 fatty acids. The omega-3 fatty acids are poly-unsaturated fats that are not made in the human body and must be consumed in one's diet.

You can add omega-3 fatty acids into your diet by eating cold-water fish (oily fish) and two types are found in salmon, trout and tuna—which contain eicosapentaenoic acid (EPA) and docosahexanoic acid (DHA). (Be aware, though, that some tuna have high levels of mercury—so read the packaging carefully.) Another omega-3 fatty acid is alphalinolenic acid (ALA), 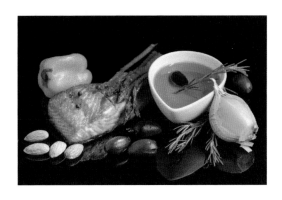 which is found commonly in flaxseed oil, fish oil, canola oil, nuts (walnuts) and soybeans. The body can convert the ALA to EPA and DHA, which are more easily used by cells. The other type of fatty acid is omega-6, which is common in breads, cereals, corn, vegetable oils and other common foods.

In the United States, the typical diet is more likely to contain the omega-6 fatty acids rather than the omega-3 fatty acids. Unfortunately, the benefits of omega-3 fatty acids are negated by the large amount of omega-6 fatty acids consumed. Researchers usually look at a 1:1 ratio when studying the amount of omega-3 to omega-6 consumed. Realistically, that ratio is closer to 1:4 for omega-3 vs. omega-6.

ALA	DHA / EPA
Walnuts	Cold water fish (salmon, bass, mackerel)
Chia, Hemp, Flax seeds	
	Grass-fed meats
Some green vegetables (broccoli, kale, brussels sprouts)	Eggs from pasteurized chickens

DHA is the most abundant omega-3 in brain cell membranes. Therefore, much of the research and trials based on omega-3 fatty acids are centered on the DHA intake. Several recent research trials were completed looking at the role of DHA in cognition and brain health. This information was compiled and presented by Julia Turner, MMSc, RD, LN and published in Generations – Journal of the American Society on Aging in an article titled "Your Brain on Food: A Nutrient-Rich Diet Can Protect Cognitive Health."

Findings indicate that six-month supplementation with 900 mg algal DHA (Algal-900) improved learning in healthy older adults with age related cognitive decline, whereas other research concluded that supplementation with 2g/d algal DHA for 18 months did not slow the rate of cognitive and functional decline in patients with mild to moderate Alzheimer's. Thus, DHA may have a preventative effect more than a treatment effect.

– Yurko-Mauo et al. (2010 study); Quinn et al. (2010 Study)

Spices
The spices that many people enjoy are high in antioxidants, which studies have shown have a positive affect on brain health.

- Oregano
- Black pepper
- Cinnamon
- Basil
- Parsley
- Ginger
- Vanilla

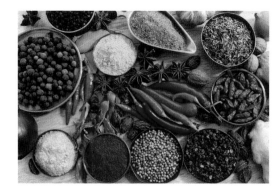

Of specific interest to researchers is the spice curcumin. Some studies have shown that the spice has the ability to clear amyloid beta plaques in mice with Alzheimer's disease. One theory is that there is a correlation with a decreased incidence of AD in the Indian population directly related to the high amount of curcumin in the diet.

Antioxidants – walnuts, berries, cloves

To understand the effectiveness of antioxidants, here's a look at why they are important: The human brain requires the most amount of oxygen in your body to fire the nerve cells and allow your body to function. However, highly reactive forms of oxygen called free radicals create chemical reactions that can damage brain cells. The brain needs antioxidants to regulate its oxygen level and to control the free radicals. These free radicals are imperative to several functions in the brain including metabolism. But, if the proportion of free radicals gets too high, then the brain cells can be damaged before your brain has time to repair them.

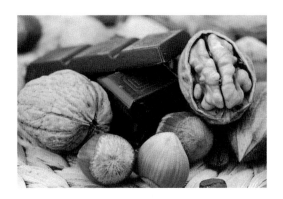

When there are more free radicals in the brain than necessary it creates what is called "Oxidative Stress" on your brain. Oxidative stress is thought to be a part of several degenerative diseases including cognitive decline, cancer, and heart disease. Therefore, the brain requires foods that have a high oxygen radical absorbance capacity (ORAC), such as pecans and walnuts.

Several studies have shown that a diet full of antioxidants leads to increased cognition, learning, awareness and brain cell growth. Recent findings demonstrate a possible link between high antioxidants and a decrease in cognitive decline.

Now, let's look at the foods with high levels of antioxidants:
• Blueberries
• Walnuts
• Chocolate (in moderation)
• Cinnamon
• Brightly colored fruits and vegetables
• Red wine (in moderation)

Vitamin B

Vitamin B plays a critical role in brain function. Vitamin B's main job is to aid in breaking down carbohydrates into sugar, blood glucose, which is the primary source of energy for all cells. Side effects of a low level of Vitamin B in the brain could include: fatigue, problems focusing, and fuzzy memory. Vitamin B is vital for the biochemical reactions in your cells, which affect the brain cell's chemicals and neurotransmitters, which are integral in the communication between your brain cells. In addition, Vitamin B aids in reducing the oxidative stress throughout your body and brain cells.

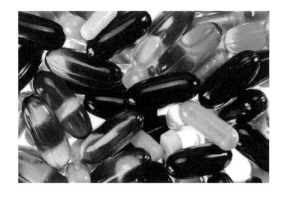

For those making a doctor's office visit to find out about any issues with memory, the first test ordered by your physician typically is for Vitamin B12 deficiency. One symptom of a Vitamin B12 deficiency is memory loss. The good news is that a Vitamin B12 deficiency, while it cannot be cured, can be treated effectively. Most multivitamins have the daily-recommended dosage of Vitamin B.

Coffee and tea

Coffee has been shown to stimulate and potentially provide some protective properties for the brain.

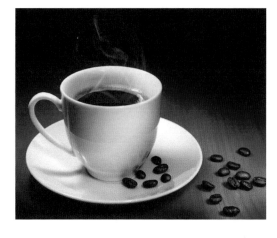

A study in Finland and Sweden a few years ago followed 1,400 people over a 20-year timeframe. The researchers found that those who drank three to five cups of coffee a day in midlife had a 65% lower chance of developing Alzheimer's disease or other forms of dementia—compared with those who drank little or no coffee. Other studies over the past several years point to additional overall health benefits of caffeine. Researchers are aiming to determine a "critical level" of caffeine needed to give protective advantages.

In a case control study last year, researchers from the University of Miami and the University of South Florida (USF) monitored the thinking processes and memory of individuals between age 65 and 80. They found that the study participants with higher levels of caffeine in their blood (mainly from drinking coffee) avoided the occurrence of AD in a two- to four-year follow-up. This also was the case of those with mild cognitive impairment. This study, which was published in the Journal of Alzheimer's Disease, offers the first direct evidence that caffeine/coffee intake may be linked to a lowered risk of dementia or a delay in its onset.

The lead author of this study (Chuanhai Cao, a neuroscientist at USF College of Pharmacy and USF Health Byrd Alzheimer's Institute) and his colleagues also authored other findings on memory impairment. They found that if aged mice—with symptoms of AD—were given the equivalent of five cups of coffee a day, it could reverse two indicators of the disease: 1) memory impairment and 2) the distinguishing protein in the brain and blood.

However, they cautioned that caffeine is a key but that it probably does not act alone. Cao and his team have reported that the caffeine likely acts together with another not yet identified ingredient in coffee to stall the Alzheimer's disease process. Other studies reveal that teas may also optimize brain function, especially green and black teas that have caffeine in them. Tea typically has half as much caffeine as coffee.

Planning a "healthy brain" diet

Having a well-balanced diet may not only help you fit into your favorite outfit, but it may also help lower your risk of age-related brain decline. In addition, it could help stave off dementia. Check out the following chart of recommended foods, vitamins and drinks for a "brain-healthy" diet:

Omega-3 Fatty Acids
Cold water fish, green vegetables ADA Guidelines - 500mg of DHA/EPA
Antioxidents
Blueberries Brightly colored fruits and vegetables
Vitamin B
Multivitamins Beef, chicken, fish Recommended 2.4 international units per day
Vitamin E
Oils (fish, olive), walnuts, spinach, broccoli
Vitamin D
Multivitamins Fish, milk Sunlight!
Coffee & Green Tea
Studies have shown that coffee and tea may decrease cognitive decline
Conclusion
Eat well-balanced meals Use spices Brightly colored fruits and vegetables Omega-3 is critical

Sources:
(http://www.alz.org/we_can_help_brain_health_maintain_your_brain.asp)
(http://www.ars.usda.gov/is/ar/archive/aug07/aging0807.htm)
(http://www.nutritionj.com/content/9/1/3)
(https://www.ibp.ucla.edu/research/GomezPinilla/publications/Diet1457.pdf)
(http://www.orac-info-portal.de/download/ORAC_R2.pdf)
(http://www.ncbi.nlm.nih.gov/pubmed/21402242)
(http://www.ncbi.nlm.nih.gov/pubmed/21045096)
(http://www.ncbi.nlm.nih.gov/pubmed/17066210)
(http://www.medicalnewstoday.com/articles/247583.php)
(http://www.ncbi.nlm.nih.gov/pubmed/18568016)
(http://www.mendeley.com/catalog/highfat-diets-insulin-resistance-declining-cognitive-function/)

CHAPTER 7

Rejuvenate Your Mind and Spirit – Music and Art Therapy

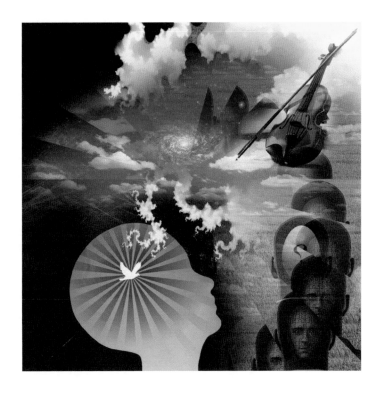

From haunting melodies to toe-tapping tunes, why is it that music seems to affect people so powerfully? Just how potent is music's effect on the brain? Over the last decade, scientists have been able to develop the technology that may provide answers to these questions. They are coming up with solid evidence that music can have a profound influence on the health of the human brain.

In fact, their research suggests that music may someday have the ability to help patients who have Alzheimer's disease, dementia, Parkinson's disease, or had a stroke.

The power of music

Music can have a profound influence on brain health, according to Elena Mannes, author of *The Power of Music*. She recently told NPR's *Talk of the Nation* that music can have a profound influence on brain health. Mannes says that current technology (such as PET scans and fMRI scans) enables researchers to look at how music affects the brain.

"Scientists believe that music uses more parts of the brain than any other functions that we perform," she says. "That's why music has so much potential to change the brain and affect the way the brain works."

"The potential of music to help people with neurological deficits is immense. Scientists believe there is some overlap of music and language in the brain," adds Mannes.

Music therapy shows promise

"Music, of course, triggers many associations in our memories," she continues. "Alzheimer's patients will respond to music long after they have lost the ability to respond to anything else,"

Recent studies showed that music therapy could help those with Alzheimer's and dementia in significant ways:
- Improves social behaviors by providing a way to interact with others
- Reduces restlessness and wandering
- Helps soothe patients, lowering their agitation levels

Whether music therapy is effective or not will depend on the individual, the quality and length of treatment, and other factors.

Making music more accessible for the elderly

The value of maintaining the mind is so important to some people like social worker Dan Cohen, that he founded a group called Music & Memory. The group brings music on iPods to elderly and infirm residents in long-term care facilities. During his visits, Cohen discovered that residents with memory loss seemed to "awaken" at the sound of the familiar music to which they may have an emotional attachment.

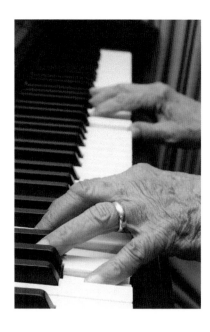

Oliver Sachs, a neurologist, explains why this might happen in HuffPost Healthy Living. "Music imprints itself on the brain deeper than any other human experience. Music evokes emotion, and emotion can bring with it memory."

Music therapy can bring back self-awareness! Recently Dan Cohen, founder of MusicandMemory.org produced a documentary movie titled "Alive Inside". This movie focuses on "Dan's journey to help those with Alzheimer's and other dementias reawaken their souls through the simple, profound experience of listening to their favorite music." This feature won the 2014 Sundance Film Festival's U.S. Documentary Audience award.

Although music therapy has been used in nursing home facilities since the 1940s, the use of iPods and other current technology makes music more accessible. Combine that with the availability of trained music therapists—and it's a powerful combination.

We would suggest creating a favorite music list. It doesn't have to be by specific artist for older music—it can be by genre, like swing, jazz or classical. Purchase an easy-to-use music player like an iPod Shuffle and select a set of headphones that the individual is comfortable wearing. Some people like headphones that cover the ears, while others prefer the ear-bud types. Put together a music library on the portable device and be sure to test the sound level before you hand over the headphones. Most individuals will enjoy sitting listening to music for several hours at a time. You might see individuals get up and dance to certain songs.

The effect of song on the mind

Singing is another musical activity that can offer a way for those with dementia, along with their caregivers, to express themselves and socialize with others in a fun and supportive group. Implicit in the fun are activities that build on the preserved memory for song and music in the brain. Even when many memories are hard to retrieve, music is especially easy to recall.

Can art therapy aid Alzheimer's patients?

Art therapy might offer individuals with dementia a way to express themselves with other forms of communication that do not rely on cognitive or verbal skills.

Some people might limit their verbal communication because they have a fear of saying the wrong thing, or they avoid contact with things they cannot understand. Sharing an interest in art with someone might be another path to communication and could be stimulating at the same time.

Arnold Bresky, MD, who calls himself a "preventive gerontologist," says art can have a positive influence on brain health. Dr. Bresky claims to have used art therapy effectively for his patients with Alzheimer's and dementia. He estimates that he has had a 70% success rate in improving the memory of his patients.

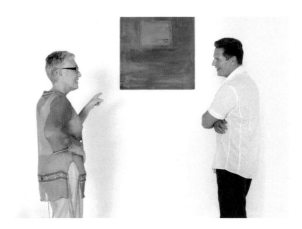

"The brain works through numbers and patterns," Dr. Bresky says. "The numbers are on the left side of your brain, the patterns are on the right side. What I'm doing is connecting the two sides."

"And we're getting the brain to grow new cells. It's called `brain plasticity.' The brain changes physically to the environment."

Art does not have to include creating something, but using art to explore ways to communicate may be helpful. A trip to a favorite art museum or special exhibit provides a platform for discussion. Standing or sitting in front of paintings or sculptures stimulates the mind. Start a discussion about describing what each one sees in the painting.

Check with your local art museum or senior center to see if there is an arts program focused on individuals with dementia. Several art programs like Memories in the Making® in southern California or The MetLife Foundation Creative Aging Libraries Project in Boston, Dallas and Miami are some good examples of using art to promote meaningful social engagement.

Sources:

(http://www.npr.org/2011/06/01/136859090/the-power-of-music-to-affect-the-brain)

(http://www.huffingtonpost.com/ronna-kaplan-ma/music-therapy_b_1749980.html)

(http://www.medscape.com/viewarticle/773401)

(http://www.arttherapyblog.com/art-therapy-seniors/art-therapy-helps-alzheimers-patients-improve-memory/#ixzz2C7YO1xTR)

CHAPTER 8

How Does Lifestyle Affect Your Brain?

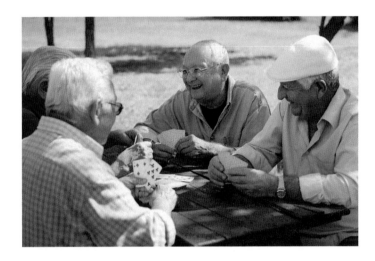

Having good friends may be good for your health—at least that's what many researchers have determined. As people age, those who stay active socially have a better chance of preserving their mental health and fending off dementia.

A study published in the American Journal of Public Health found that maintaining close relationships and engaging with others in large social networks are key factors in keeping the brain healthier. Such studies have not yet pinpointed what happens in the brain to bring about these positive results.

The study, which involved over 2,200 older women, found that those who had bigger social networks were 26% less prone to developing dementia than those with smaller ones. The women who enjoyed everyday contact with friends and family members actually reduced their risk of Alzheimer's or other forms of dementia by nearly 50%.

Boost brain health through socializing

Studies such as these validate the recommendation that older adults who stay active with others can make a difference in their brain's health. Social engagements also tend to encourage healthy behaviors, such as getting involved in a bowling league or a daily walking group.

Of course, exercise goes hand-in-hand with socialization in helping to delay pathological changes in the brain that may lead to cognitive impairment. The first clinical trial showing that physical workouts might improve cognitive function among people with mild impairment was published in the Journal of the American Medical Association. It turns out that exercise, especially when paired with socializing, may help boost the formation of brain synapses and nerve cells—to help increase the circulation of blood in the brain.

The Mayo Clinic Alzheimer's Research Center also concurs that exercise combined with socialization boosts brain health. Engaging in physical, intellectual and social activities together with eating heart-healthy foods all coordinate to maintain your brain.

Access to the Internet and cellular networks make it possible for anyone anywhere to have face-to-face or voice-to-voice real time contact. Real time video allows users to communicate face-to-face with a simple technology interface. Skype™, Google Voice and FaceTime are examples of services that can easily connect friends and family. The simplicity and accessibility of services like Skype™ can increase the likelihood that an older adult receives the regular motivation and reinforcement necessary 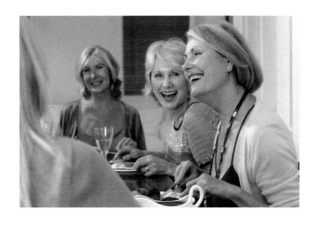 to stick with an exercise regimen that can delay the onset of AD. Access via these communication tools enables individuals living in rural areas to keep socially active and in touch with family members.

Stay independent and active with others

Many neurologists encourage individuals to remain as independent as possible as they age. And we know many older adults live alone. It is very important to not become isolated. Here are some important tips for stimulating your brain:

- Hobbies – Classes
- Social Activities, senior centers, book clubs, TV discussions
- Challenge yourself, do tasks that require thinking
- Use your non-dominant hand to perform simple tasks
    Brushing your teeth

> Combing your hair
> Buttoning your shirt
> Opening lids

- Orientation of time and place
- Read the paper
- Discuss current events, celebrate holidays and birthdays
- Reminiscence therapy
- Keep a Journal
- Write your biography
- Set GOALS!
  > 2 weeks, one month,
  > Update the goals, celebrate the accomplishments
  > Keep it in a central location
- Behavioral therapy
- Exercise

Get enough ZZZs

Set a regular sleeping schedule. You need 7 to 8 hours of sleep each night to regenerate your brain cells. Your brain performs its "housekeeping" functions while you sleep in addition to storing memories. Many older adults do not get enough sleep at night, which can cause daytime sleepiness. To help you sleep better these tips may be helpful:

- Make sure your bedroom is dark and quiet and not too warm
- Adjust your bedtimes, go to bed when you feel tired and get up at the same time each day
- Turn off the TV at least 1 hour before going to bed
- Wind down before bed by taking a bath or listening to soft music or reading

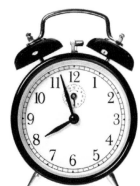

During the night, your sleep follows a predictable pattern, moving back and forth between deep restorative sleep and more alert stages and dreaming known as REM sleep. Together, the stages of REM and non-REM sleep form a complete sleep cycle. Each cycle typically lasts about 90 minutes and repeats four to six times over the course of a night.

The amount of time you spend in each stage of sleep changes as the night progresses. For example, most deep sleep occurs in the first half of the night. Later in the night, your REM sleep stages become longer, alternating with lighter sleep. This is why if you are sensitive to waking in the middle of the night, it is probably in the early morning hours, not immediately after going to bed.

Here is some good advice if you are having a hard time getting up with your alarm goes off!

Even if you've enjoyed a full night's sleep, getting out of bed can be difficult if your alarm goes off when you are in the middle of deep sleep. If you want to make mornings less painful—or if you know you only have a limited time for sleep—try setting a wake-up time that's a multiple of 90 minutes, the length of the average sleep cycle. For example, if you go to bed at 10 p.m., set your alarm for 5:30, giving you a total of 7 ½ hours of sleep, instead of 6:00 or 6:30. You may feel more refreshed at 5:30 than with another 30 to 60 minutes of sleep because you're getting up at the end of a sleep cycle when your body and brain are already close to wakefulness.

Sources:
(http://ajph.aphapublications.org/doi/abs/10.2105/AJPH.2007.115923)
(http://jama.jamanetwork.com/article.aspx?articleid=199487)
(http://www.healthcommunities.com/healthy-aging/healthy-living-tips-70s-
     older-elderly.shtml)

CHAPTER 9

Why Your Mind Matters

Interview with Dr. Dougherty

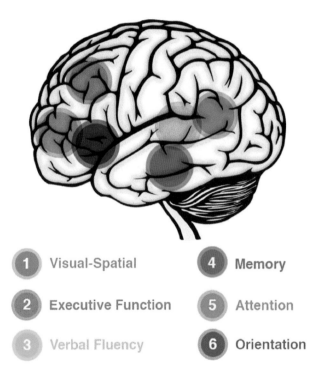

1	Visual-Spatial		4	Memory
2	Executive Function		5	Attention
3	Verbal Fluency		6	Orientation

A critical part of being human is having a healthy mind—with its cognitive functions ranging from memory to decision-making. The mind has an amazing capacity to learn new things, remember complicated events in our environment, and make complex decisions. It gives us access to executive function in a way that's very powerful.

Get on the path to better brain health!
Our ultimate goal in introducing the COGselftest to the public and providing further insights in this book is to show why *your mind matters*. We have offered suggestions on what you can do to protect your brain health, and now the rest is up to you.

We can't overemphasize the importance of assessing your brain health. Becoming aware of the various tests available is essential—so that you can take steps early enough to keep your gray matter as healthy as possible.

Soon, routine cognitive testing will become as widespread as testing for cholesterol or heart disease and become a regular part of our overall health evaluation—just as yearly mammograms have been emphasized throughout the United States.

You've taken the first step in caring about the future of your brain. After all, it's not just about you—the health of your brain affects everyone in your family and has a great impact on our society. The cost of care for Alzheimer's patients in the United States for families and society is between $157 billion to $215 billion a year, according to a study by the non-profit RAND Corp. The largest expense is not the medical treatments or drugs, but the care needed to get people with dementia through daily routines.

Questions and Answers (about Why Your Mind Matters)

The following is an interview with Dr. John Dougherty, Jr., and Andrew Dougherty, Co-founders of Medical Interactive Education, LLC, *by Laura Carlson, Health and Science Writer*

Q1 – How does Medinteract intend to improve awareness of brain health across the United States, and then globally?

A1 – Dr. D: The human brain is capable of objective reasoning. By increasing awareness of the brain's capacity and need to protect its functioning, it will allow us to focus on brain health in the way our society has dealt with heart problems, hypertension and cancer. By spreading this awareness, it gives people better tools for taking a proactive approach to their brain health.

Andrew: We're living longer—the average life expectancy in 1930 was 60 and today a typical American's life expectancy is 78. And with longer life comes an increased risk of AD and other forms of dementia. We need to take a personal approach to help delay the onset of these diseases and increase the years in which we live in good health.

It is important to address cognitive impairment early. You can reduce the population of Alzheimer's patients [within the United States] by the [size of the] metropolitan population of Atlanta just by delaying the onset. We have some good treatment options available now, but they can only be effective if we diagnose the disease early—when treatment options are most effective."

Q2 – How does the COGselftest compare to other top cognitive health assessments?

A2 – Dr. D: First, it's computer-based and accessible through the Internet. Second, it evaluates cognition in the sense that it measures multiple cognitive domains—memory, executive function, visual-spatial, verbal fluency, attention and orientation. It has a score reflecting one's individual cognitive abilities. You can track the results over time. By screening at regular intervals, we can make inroads in delaying the onset of Alzheimer's or other forms of dementia.

Andrew: You can take the **COGselftest** at home—or anywhere you have access to the Internet. You can take charge of your brain health using this Better Brain Health book and if you are concerned with your memory or your results, you can choose to take the results of the test to your physician.

Q3- How accurate is the COGselftest? How was it evaluated for effectiveness?

A3 – Andrew: It is 96 percent accurate. We have a database of 3,500 tests that include a normal control group, one with mild cognitive impairment and others with moderate to severe AD and other forms of dementia. Using this database, we compare it to other tests and physician's diagnoses to measure accuracy. The 96 percent is about the sensitivity to cognitive impairment. The specificity is approximately 91 percent in determining what type of dementia. Our validation article was published in the Journal of Alzheimer's Disease in April 2010. We continue to be active in the area of developing additional cognitive tests.

Q4 – What do you feel are the best exercises to maintain brain fitness?

A4 – Dr. D: Two things are important. We now recognize that physical exercise is a very significant factor in improving memory and overall brain health. How strenuous should that physical activity be? We're not sure yet. We are continuing to research specific exercise programs. It may not just be that it improves our cardiovascular status, but that exercise changes the protein in the brain itself.

Andrew: Some studies have suggested we exercise our brain by doing tasks that affect brain capacity. Games and puzzles are helpful and could be very important. However, you need to be sure that you do not become so good at a game or puzzle, crossword puzzles for example, because then you lose the benefit of exercising the brain. It is important to switch around so that you're learning something new. Recent studies have shown cognitive benefits from playing games on the computer.

It's also very important to increase social activities. You're requiring your brain to react to different cues. For example, I need to adjust my conversation when I see that someone is sad or angry. So you're not doing the same tasks every time. You're challenging yourself on a daily basis.

So maintaining and increasing one's social experience is an integral part of your overall brain health. Exercise the body, exercise the mind, and be socially active.

Q5 – You talked about objective memory tests earlier. What's the difference between "objective memory" test scores and "subjective" ones?

A5 – Dr. D: 'Objective' has a statistical basis to it—like COGselftest. 'Subjective' is just saying their condition improves. AD patients have a condition called anasognosia, in which they say they're OK, but when testing them objectively they have a very significant brain health issue that they don't recognize.

After someone takes a COGselftest, you may see that they have a problem. For instance, they say, "I've been driving for 40 years. I'm a great driver. Then they may get lost easily; but they don't recognize that this is a cognitive problem that is worsening.

Q6 – What are some basic memory training skills that can help a person who suspects he or she has mild cognitive impairment?

A6 – Dr. D.: We believe MCI may be an early form of AD. Some medications that we suggest for AD may slow down the progression of MCI and prevent it from converting to AD. About 10 to 15 percent of those with MCI convert to AD each year. Some 20 percent can actually improve. It's a mixed condition. Sometimes it's anxiety and/or depression that can cause issues with memory and cognition. We really have pretty effective treatment for depression. It's so critical to do objective testing like doing the COGselftest. A lot of people with depression complain bitterly about their memory, but it may just be depression or anxiety.

Q7- We've all heard the famed expression, "Use it or lose it." What do you suggest are some of the best ways to train your brain?

A7 – Andrew: The concept that we can only make significant leaps in our brain development while we are young is not only out-dated but completely false. It's important to continue to challenge our brains. For instance, learning how to use a new mobile phone or other computer device is stimulating to the brain. The idea that learning stops when we end school is outdated. We must continue to challenge ourselves to learn new things and create new memories!

Dr. D.: By and large for elderly people—just being old does not necessarily cause a problem with memory. The idea of it being part of normal aging is no longer valid. The idea that we can create new brain cells as we continue to learn is valid. Exercise and cognitive training can grow new neurons. As an example I had one patient take charge of their brain health by enrolling in classes at the local university to learn a new language. We have a university here that has credited courses and individual classes geared to the aging population.

Q8 – For people who have been referred to a neurologist for further testing, what can they expect first?

A8 – Dr. D.: The first and most critical feature is a good history. Something I've developed is a "neurocognitive review of systems." I ask questions such as, "Do you repeat yourself?" These reviews can be given in an easy and very non-traumatic way. I'm looking for an objective evaluation of their health. I also have ways to ask and evaluate their personal and social activities.

I also do certain blood tests looking for low thyroid, B-12 deficiencies, as both can cause problems with memory or cognition. I usually obtain one set of structural and functional imaging studies.

Q9 – What 's the difference between MRI and PET scans?

A9 – Dr. D.: The MRI scan displays the structural integrity of the brain. A MRI scan takes an excellent visual photo – and the interpreting physician can look for conditions like mini-strokes or key structural changes that are known to be associated with dementia. Brain imaging with MRI and PET/CT differentiates AD from other types of dementia.

A PET scan or PET/CT scan looks at the function (metabolic activity) within the brain. Physicians interpreting PET scans look for abnormal patterns of uptake in certain areas of the brain that correspond with AD or other types of dementia.

The thing that's really going to revolutionize this diagnostic method is something that attaches to the beta amyloid protein in the brain. Now, with new amyloid tracers recently approved by the FDA, we have a way to identify beta amyloid plaques in the brain.

This new agent will be able to help us measure the response to medication that we might use for treatment and many clinical trials are underway. It looks like people who are predisposed may have proteins in their brain that can be measured years in advance of any clinical symptoms. But it raises some ethical questions. Do you really want to know? Can it make a difference in your medical future? The answer is that it can make a difference so that you can get involved in these things that can make a difference.

Q10 - What about APOE Testing? Please define this type of testing and its status.

A10 – Dr. D.: APOE is the genetic material that increases the probability that you may get AD. It's not been advocated in the past since it has not been well developed or very accurate. The thing that may change that… is the ability to image the beta amyloid proteins in the brain itself.

Q11–What if a family member with dementia starts taking a prescribed medication for the disease and begins having side-effects? Are there alternatives?

A11 – Dr. D.: With one specific medication, some people may develop nausea or vomiting. However, there are alternatives that cause very few gastrointestinal problems by using different dosages or drug delivery methods. We have three or four meds we use routinely, so that if you adjust the dose or frequency, most people can tolerate the treatment we recommend.

Q12- What can you try to do to empower the patient and the family?

A12 - Dr. D: To take over the care and address the things I tell them about in a really proactive and energetic way so they can attack this disease.

It's important to have openness about it. Tell your friends, tell your family so they can participate in the management. Look at one of our sports' heroes, Pat Summitt. Her teams won eight national championships. She's talking openly about it, on NPR and other media channels. She's talking about her life and the experience of addressing AD. We're beginning a revolution in the management and treatment of AD.

Andrew: You have to take a personalized approach to this. For example, I'm not going to just tell you to walk a mile a week. I want you to do things that interest you. I want you to eat healthy—but of the foods that you like. It takes 28 days for a lifestyle change to become a habit. Our challenge is to get you through those 28 days. We have to create a plan that is customized to you.

Dr. D: I'll give you an example of that. I had a patient who is a retired physicist, and he had a lot of technical hobbies in the past. So he took up photography, which can be a little simpler than quadratic equations. He was telling me that he plans to go with a group to Africa this summer and take pictures of wild animals. What an opportunity for him to engage his cognitive capacity! It's something that will stimulate his mind in a way he hadn't ever done in the past.

Q13 – Please tell us your thoughts about support groups for families and their loved ones with Alzheimer's disease or dementia?

A13 – Dr. D.: Education of the family and the patient himself or herself is so important. We have local support groups in Knoxville. It's important to find a group in your community (or start a group if there is not one) because the group dynamic provides support to the caregiver as well as the individual affected with dementia.

Q14 – What have you discovered about the role of those who care for people with AD or other form of dementia?

A14 - Dr. D.: One of the most important 'treatments' for AD is to support the caregiver because quite often that person can become depressed or burdened with additional stress. I always tell the caregiver that they're doing a great job, They're real heroes.

Andrew: Look for more Q&A sessions coming to the blog on CognitiveTest. com, and in updates to the Better Brain Health book. Our goal is to keep you informed about medical and science news in addition to helping you understand how these updates are impacting treatments for dementia.

CHAPTER 10

Resources and Updates

"The woman I've been married to for 29 years—the mother of my children, the one I intended to travel around the world with after the kids were all set—doesn't even know me when I come in to visit her."

- Alan Holbrook, spouse of Alzheimer's patient
from "I Am Not Alone"—courtesy alz.org

What would you do if your spouse, family member, friend or even you developed dementia? Are you aware of how or where to find medical advice and assistance, and what types of medications may be available for someone with dementia? How much would care cost if your loved one (or you) needs to stay in a memory care facility? Do you know how long your finances would last? Do you know the type of assistance programs available in your community or what Government programs might be available? If you need help, do you know what resources are offered?

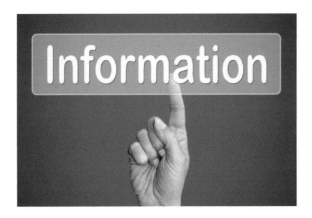

It is important to gather information from reliable and credible sources. Fortunately there is a heightened awareness and focus on brain science related to all neurological diseases, particularly dementia. Keep informed by using our Blog and ask Dr. Dougherty forums.

(http://www.cognitivetest.com/blog/)

In this chapter, you'll find important information that will help you to answer these important questions.

AD symptoms vs. normal aging

At this point, you now realize that Alzheimer's disease is much more than simple forgetfulness.

Learn more about the symptoms:

Early symptoms of AD	Normal age-related changes
Problems recalling recent events	Some issues recalling past events
Poor judgment and decision-making ability	Making a silly choice every so often
Difficulty managing a budget	Forgetting to make a payment
Losing track of the season	Not recalling what day it is, then remembering later
Problems carrying on a conversation; repeating a question or story over and over not realizing they've asked the question before	Occasionally unable to think of which word to use; remember when you repeat a question
Putting things away, and then being unable to recall where you put them	Losing things from time to time
Changes in mood and personality, inappropriate social behavior	Developing specific ways of doing things, and getting upset if the routine is changed
Withdrawing from socializing	Sometimes feeling fatigued about social obligations
Encountering new problems with speech	Sometimes having difficulty finding the right word
Difficulty understanding visuals	Problems with vision due to age-related eye issues
Problems finishing familiar tasks	Needing help with technical settings sometimes

Remember, you can choose to take the COGselftest results to your personal care physician, who will determine whether you need further testing.

Physician Visit – getting prepared:

If you are going to visit your personal care physician or take a loved one to visit their personal care physician for issues related to cognitive changes, what do you need to **prepare** for that particular visit?

- Be sure to let the physician's staff know this appointment is about a possible cognitive issue so if there are any restrictions you might have to follow for lab work or other tests you are prepared.
- Write down your concerns and symptoms because your physician is going to want to know details about what is causing your concern. Make notes about examples of lapses in memory or behavior changes you or a loved one have noticed.
- Bring someone with you to the appointment. Your physician will want to confirm these changes are noticed by others.
- Be sure to write out a list of all your medications, even over-the-counter drugs, vitamins and/or supplements, how much you are taking and when you are taking them. *(Sometimes it is easier to take all the bottles to the office visit)*
- Prepare a list of questions you want to ask your physician.

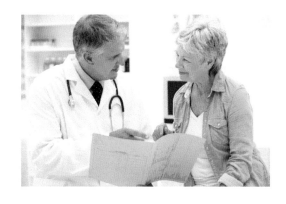

What can you expect from your physician visit?

Your physician will ask you questions about any memory lapses; activities you perform; have you had previous head injuries; are you sad or anxious; do you get lost; how is your driving; do you drink alcohol, how much; do you have trouble walking or have you noticed any trembling; has anyone in your family had memory problems or ever been diagnosed with a dementia like Alzheimer's disease.

- Your physician will most likely want to perform lab tests to rule out causes of memory loss or cognitive changes like thyroid disease or vitamin deficiencies.
- Your physician may conduct mental status tests or refer you to a neurologist for a detailed series of neuropsychological tests.
- Your physician will check your muscle tone, strength, reflexes, walking, balance, and coordination and ask about your sight and hearing.
- Your physician may order brain-imaging studies like CT, MRI or PET scans.

CT Scan – an imaging study used to rule out tumors, head injuries and strokes.

MRI Scan – an imaging study also used to rule out conditions like tumors, head injuries or strokes; MRI is also used to identify anatomic changes within certain areas of the brain associated with dementias like Alzheimer's disease.

FDG PET Scan – an imaging study used to show overall metabolic activity in various regions of the brain. This scan can identify which parts of the brain aren't functioning well and is often used to differentiate frontotemporal dementia from Alzheimer's disease.

Amyloid PET Scan – an imaging study used to detect beta-amyloid deposits in the brain. Appropriateness criteria were recently published and physicians are just now beginning to understand when it is appropriate to order this scan. The scan is widely used in clinical trials and physicians are beginning to use it in routine clinical practice.

If you are referred to a neurologist or neuropsychologist for further testing it is because your personal care physician would like you to have a more extensive assessment of your cognitive changes. Neuropsychological testing will take several hours and will provide additional, comprehensive information on your mental function.

What treatments or drugs are available?

There are several prescription drugs available to treat individuals diagnosed with Alzheimer's disease. These drugs are used to treat cognitive symptoms. Cholinesterase inhibitors are used in mild to moderate Alzheimer's disease. Cholinesterase inhibitors include Aricept (donepezil), Razadyne (galantamine) and Exelon (rivastigmine). Treatment for moderate to severe Alzheimer's disease is done using a medication known as Namenda (memantine). Sometimes a cholinesterase inhibitor is given in combination with memantine.

This Alzheimer's disease Medications Fact Sheet was updated in January 2014. This document is also available in Spanish.

http://www.nia.nih.gov/alzheimers/publication/alzheimers-disease-medications-fact-sheet

FDA update

In March 2013, The New England Journal of Medicine reported that the U.S. Food and Drug Administration might ease its guidelines for approving certain medications for treating Alzheimer's disease.

The FDA's proposal to loosen its guidelines has the potential to help millions of people who may be at risk for developing AD. It could make it easier for those patients with symptoms of early onset AD to get access to medications that help stave off the disease. Plus, this proposed change in guidelines could facilitate the testing and approval of drugs for researchers and pharmaceutical companies.

(http://www.nejm.org/doi/full/10.1056/NEJMp1302513?query=featured_ home&)

Clinical trials

It might be hard to wrap your head around the term "clinical trail". We often relate clinical trial to cancer or heart disease, but there are many clinical trials focused on Alzheimer's disease that are testing new drugs and lifestyle changes. Volunteers are needed and it is very easy to find information on a trial that might be in your area.

Find Alzheimer's disease and Related Clinical Trials through the National Institute on Aging – National Institute on Health – select your state and review new and ongoing trials at:
(http://www.nia.nih.gov/alzheimers/clinical-trials)

The Alzheimer's Prevention Registry – a very good resource to find Alzheimer's prevention studies and trials taking place near you:
(http://www.endalznow.org/study-opportunities)

Two of the longest running trials are the DIAN trial and the ADNI trial.

DIAN Study – Dominantly Inherited Alzheimer Network – studying individuals with early onset Alzheimer's disease:
(http://www.dian-exr.org/)

ADNI – Alzheimer's Disease Neuroimaging Initiative – studying all phases of Alzheimer's disease:
(http://www.adni-info.org/)

Another important trail recently got underway – the A4 study – Anti-Amyloid Treatment in Asymptomatic Alzheimer's – check it out at:
(http://a4study.org/)

The Alzheimer's Association has a trial match service that can connect individuals with current trials.

(http://www.alz.org/research/clinical_trials/find_clinical_trials_
trialmatch.asp)

RESOURCES

Having a plan in place for caring for yourself or a loved one with dementia is highly recommended—so that it's available in case you need it. There are many places to turn for help. We have come across many valuable resources over these recent years. Although we do not endorse any specific products, services or organizations, we are providing links to documents, web sites, articles and organizations we feel are helpful and informative. Please feel free to ask about any type of resource at **info@cognitivetest.com** We will check our extensive data bank and get back with you.

LEGAL MATTERS

The Essentials – Legal Matters from the MetLife Mature Market Institute Answers all questions related to legal matters from wills to durable power of attorney to advance directives.
   (https://www.metlife.com/assets/cao/mmi/publications/essentials/mmi-
   legal-matters-essentials.pdf)

Alzheimer's Disease Education and Referral Center legal and financial planning fact sheet
   (http://www.nia.nih.gov/alzheimers/publication/legal-and-financial-
   planning-people-alzheimers-disease-fact-sheet)

SSI – Compassionate Allowances for individuals with Early Onset Alzheimer's Disease & Related Dementias – the Social Security Administration has added early-onset Alzheimer's disease as one of the conditions that qualify for Compassionate Allowance Program.
   (https://secure.ssa.gov/apps10/poms.nsf/lnx/0423022385)

CARE OPTIONS OUTSIDE THE HOME

Many national and local organizations offer updates and recommendations on how to address assisted living and long-term care – including how to pay for these services.
   Helpguide.org has published a helpful resource guide on assisted living and

we have also included a link to the Medicare.gov site on "Paying for Long-Term Care".

(http://www.helpguide.org/elder/assisted_living_facilities.htm)
(http://longtermcare.gov/medicare-medicaid-more/medicare)

The Centers for Medicare and Medicaid Services (CMS) – primarily through Medicaid – provides coverage for certain services related to dementia care. Nursing facilities are routinely inspected and evaluated based on strict quality measures. Please be sure to look at the quality rating of a facility you might be considering. Here are links to the appropriate resource sections.

(http://www.cms.gov/Medicare/Provider-Enrollment-and-Certification/
CertificationandComplianc/FSQRS.html)

(http://www.medicaid.gov/Medicaid-CHIP-Program-Information/By-
Topics/Delivery-Systems/Institutional-Care/Nursing-Facilities-NF.html
CertificationandComplianc/FSQRS.html)

(http://www.medicaid.gov/Medicaid-CHIP-Program-Information/By-
Topics/Delivery-Systems/Institutional-Care/Nursing-Facilities-NF.html)

MISCELLANEOUS RESOURCES

Excellent video sessions:
Visualmd – What is Alzheimer's disease – this 12 part series takes you through the amazing journey of the disease – from diagnosis through all the phases.

(http://www.thevisualmd.com/interactives
php?idu=1033607531&idc=1367&cw=3)

Alzheimer's Disease Education and Referral Center – video "Inside the Brain – Unraveling the Mystery of Alzheimer's disease"

(http://www.nia.nih.gov/alzheimers/alzheimers-disease-video)

Mild Cognitive Impairment:
Information for individuals, families and caregivers

(http://www.caregiver.org/caregiver/jsp/content_node.jsp?nodeid=2501)

Frontotemporal Disorders:
Information for individuals, families and caregivers

(http://www.nia.nih.gov/sites/default/files/frontotemporal_disorders_
information_for_patients_families_and_caregivers_0.pdf)

Lewy body dementia:

Information and resources for individuals, families and caregivers
(http://www.lbda.org/)

All of this information and associated links are available at:
CognitiveTest.com/blog under the Resources Tab – Better Brain Health Book
Links.

Glossary

Alzheimer's Disease (AD) – AD is a degenerative brain disease that is the most common form of dementia, accounting for 60 to 70% of all dementia cases. AD is characterized by progressive memory loss, impaired thinking, disorientation, and changes in personality and mood.

Amyloid Plaques– Also referred to as beta-amyloid; these protein fragments are found naturally in the brain, but when they aggregate (clump together) into amyloid plaques they block nerve cells from signaling. Beta amyloid plaques are a characteristic feature of AD pathology. Beta-amyloid plaques are also found in the brains of individuals without Alzheimer's disease.

Dementia – Dementia is an umbrella term describing a group of symptoms that include memory loss, language difficulties, and changes in attention and problem solving. The most common type of dementia is Alzheimer's disease. Dementia is not a normal part of aging.

Dementia with Lewy Bodies – (DLB) DLB is a type of progressive dementia that leads to a decline in thinking, reasoning and independent functions. DLB may be the 3rd most common cause of dementia after AD and vascular dementia. DLB is often associated with movement symptoms like hunched posture, rigid muscles, shuffling walk, frequent unexplained falls and trouble initiating movement.

Frontotemporal Dementia – (FTD) FTD is a form of dementia affecting the frontal and temporal lobes. FTD types are placed in two basic clinical groups. The first group is defined by behavior and personality changes – this group includes Pick's disease. The second group is characterized by progressive disruption in verbal and written skills or naming and understanding meaning. Memory and other cognitive functions remain relatively unaffected. FTD is a less common form of dementia and usually occurs at a younger age.

Magnetic Resonance Imaging – (MRI) MRI scans are produced using a MRI scanner. The MRI scan will show structural and volumetric changes that occur in neurodegenerative diseases. MRI scans are performed to identify changes in certain areas of the brain known to be associated with different types of dementia and will also show if structural abnormalities are present (tumor; AVN; normal pressure hydrocephalous) or if there are changes associated with stroke or altered blood supply.

Mild Cognitive Impairment – (MCI) An individual with MCI will have problems with memory, language or other mental functions that are severe enough to be noticeable to themselves or to other people and to show up on cognitive tests. Most individuals diagnosed with MCI can still carry out routine day-to-day activities. Individuals with MCI have an increased risk of developing Alzheimer's disease over the next several years, particularly when their main problem is memory loss.

Neuroplasticity – A term used to describe adaptive changes in the function and/or structure of nerve cells or groups of nerve cells in response to changes in patterns of their use. Your brain has the ability to form new neural connections throughout life.

Positron Emission Tomography – (PET) PET scans are produced using a PET scanner or PET/CT scanner. A PET scan is performed to look at the brain's metabolic function. PET scans performed with the tracer **FDG** measure glucose metabolism. Certain areas of the brain associated with dementia will show decreased metabolic activity. PET scans performed with an amyloid plaque tracer will identify the presence of beta-amyloid plaques associated with Alzheimer's disease.

Tau (neurofibrillary tangles) – The tau protein plays a vital role in maintaining the health of nerve cells. In Alzheimer's disease tau tends to accumulate into harmful structures called neurofibrillary tangles. These tangles cause the death of the nerve cell.

Vascular Dementia – Vascular dementia is characterized by a decline in thinking skills caused by conditions that block or reduce blood flow to the brain. Vascular dementia is the 2nd most common form of dementia after Alzheimer's disease and according to the latest data, it is common to have vascular dementia in combination with other types of dementia like Alzheimer's disease.

About the Authors

John H. Dougherty, Jr., MD, is a recognized leader in the evaluation, treatment and management of patients with memory loss. He has spent more than 25 years in neurology, with a focus on Alzheimer's disease and dementia. In 2002, he developed the first online test for physicians to screen patients for symptoms of Alzheimer's and other forms of dementia. Recently, he introduced the COGselftest, an exciting new version of this online assessment—for the general public.

In 2004, he co-founded Medical Interactive Education (Medinteract), a health education organization that provides the latest research and information about brain wellness. Dr. Dougherty is the Medical Director of the Cole Neuroscience Center (Memory Disorder Program) at the University of Tennessee Medical Center in Knoxville. He has extensive clinical experience and has held varied leadership roles in the medical field.

Dr. Dougherty has served as Co-director of the Brain and Spine Institute at the UT Medical Center and today is an Assistant Professor of Medicine in neurology at UT. Over the past decade he has published numerous articles on dementia and Alzheimer's disease. Dr. Dougherty and his associates see more than 3,000 patients with cognitive impairment annually and are involved in multiple clinical trials.

Dr. Dougherty earned his undergraduate degree at the University of North Carolina and his medical degree from the University of Tennessee Medical School in Memphis. He trained in neurology at Cornell University New York Hospital and completed a two-year fellowship at Cornell in cerebrovascular disease.

Andrew Dougherty is Co-founder of Medinteract and the COGselftest. He studied finance and information systems at Tulane University and received his MBA.with concentrations both in finance and innovation/entrepreneurship from the University of Tennessee at Knoxville.

Mr. Dougherty is a consultant for a national venture capital fund, assisting in developing financial models, business plans, and market strategies. He has in-depth experience working with healthcare-related startup companies and with other organizations in multiple industries.

In addition, Mr. Dougherty developed and implemented the plan for marketing the COGselftest, a computer-based cognitive screening test. Andrew started his research and interest in Alzheimer's disease by volunteering at the Alzheimer's Association adult daycare program. He then went on to work in the Brain Bank at the University of Tennessee, researching the epidemiology of Alzheimer's disease. An in-demand public speaker, Mr. Dougherty has given numerous talks throughout the Knoxville community on the screening and prevention of Alzheimer's disease.

Sue Buckley Halliday, CNMT, is President and Co-founder of MI-COG, LLC. (www.CognitiveTest.com). She is also the Principal at AHR Memory, a resource for individuals, physicians, caregivers and others who are seeking further information on brain health, early memory loss and dementia.

Ms. Halliday studied radiologic technology at the University of Texas Medical Branch at Galveston and Nuclear Medicine Technology at Baylor University Medical Center, Dallas. Her career began as a technologist and progressed into different radiology management roles, including responsibility for billing and collections.

With over 25 years experience in the management of medical practices and business offices, Ms. Halliday has worked at organizations ranging from Baylor University Medical Center and Maxum Health Corp to US Oncology. During this time, she discovered how critical it is to understand and participate in the development of government and private payor coverage as well as payment policy development.

Active in local and national organizations, Ms. Halliday is interested in those focused on creating coverage guidelines and payment policies for amyloid PET scans and is often an invited speaker at regional and national society meetings. She has written and co-authored several articles on PET imaging and continues to be a strong advocate for expanding diagnostic services.

She recently completed her Certificate in Gerontology

Contributors:

Walker Buckley, Chief Development Officer at MI-COG, LLC (CognitiveTest.com), comes with a wealth of marketing and digital experience. Over the past decade Mr. Buckley was a Senior Account Executive with TimeWarner, CBS Radio and Clear Channel Communications where he conceived, sold and orchestrated onsite and online campaigns for agencies and national clients. Mr. Buckley earned a BA in Communication and Advertising from The University of Texas at Arlington.

Laura Carlson, Founder of Alpha Marketing, is an award-winning writer in healthcare and higher education. She has served as a communications specialist and senior writer at organizations such as Kaiser Permanente, UCLA Health System and the California Institute of Technology (Caltech).

Ms. Carlson also has been a writer for multinational companies in New York and Los Angeles, interviewing business people from all walks of life. She has done extensive volunteer work at assisted living and memory care facilities. Her mother passed away with Lewy Body dementia, and so Ms. Carlson is familiar with the joys and challenges of caring for a loved one with cognitive health issues.

Journal of Alzheimer's Disease 20 (2010) 185–195
DOI 10.3233/JAD-2010-1354
IOS Press

The Computerized Self Test (CST): An Interactive, Internet Accessible Cognitive Screening Test For Dementia

John H. Dougherty Jr.[a], Rex L. Cannon[a,b,*], Christopher R. Nicholas[a,c], Lorin Hall[a], Felicia Hare[a], Erika Carr[a,d], Andrew Dougherty[e], Jennifer Janowitz[a] and Justin Arunthamakun[a,f]

[a]Cole Neuroscience Center, Memory Disorder Clinic, University of Tennessee Medical Center, Knoxville, TN, USA
[b]Biological Psychology and Neuroscience Laboratory, Department of Psychology, University of Tennessee, Knoxville, TN, USA
[c]Clinical Psychology Program, Department of Psychology, University of Tennessee, Knoxville, TN, USA
[d]Counseling Psychology Program, Department of Psychology, University of Tennessee, Knoxville, TN, USA
[e]Medical Interactive Education, LLC, Knoxville, TN, USA
[f]Neuroscience, Financial Economics, Biology, Vanderbilt University, Nashville, TN, USA

Accepted 8 December 2009

Abstract. The computer self test (CST) is an interactive, internet-based instrument designed to assess functional cognitive domains impaired by Alzheimer's disease (AD) and mild cognitive impairment (MCI). This study consisted of 215 total subjects with a mean age of 75.24. The 84 cognitively impaired patients (excluding patients diagnosed as MCI) met all criteria set forth by NINCDS/ADRDA for the diagnosis of AD. Control participants consisted of 104 age-matched individuals who were cognitively unimpaired. All patients completed the CST prior to other routine neurocognitive procedures. The CST accurately classified 96% of the cognitively impaired individuals as compared to controls, while the Mini-Mental Status Examination (MMSE) accurately classified 71% and the Mini-Cog 69% in the same respect. In addition, the CST accurately classified 91% of the six experimental groups (control, MCI, early AD, mild to moderate, moderate to severe, and severe) as compared to 54% for the MMSE and 48% for the Mini-Cog. In conclusions, the CST demonstrates a high degree of sensitivity and specificity and is capable of accurately identifying cognitive impairment in patients with variable degrees of cognitive abnormality. This interactive internet-based cognitive screening tool may aid in early detection of cognitive impairment in the primary care setting. The ease of use and interpretation may also provide the means to obtain an accurate baseline from which to monitor cognitive changes over time.

Keywords: Alzheimer's disease, computerized cognitive screening, dementia, mild cognitive impairment

INTRODUCTION

In its earliest stages, Alzheimer's disease (AD) may include cognitive impairments in any single or multi-ple cognitive domains, including: memory, verbal fluency, orientation, visuospatial organization, executive functions, attention, and cognitive processing speed. Deficits in awareness (anosognosia) and spontaneity (affect) are also observed [1,2]. Given the insidious onset of these symptoms, early detection in the primary care setting would be an important venue to facilitate available medications that have been shown to more effectively slow the progression of AD when adminis-

*Correspondence to: Rex Cannon, Cole Neuroscience Center, University of Tennessee Medical Center, 1928 Alcoa Highway, Medical Building B, Suite 102, Knoxville, TN 37920, USA. Tel.: +1 865 300 4983; E-mail: rcannon2@utk.edu.

tered in its early stages [3–5].

Current data suggest that 60% of the patients with AD are not diagnosed in the primary care setting [6]. To date, there is debate over the most practical way to assess early symptoms in AD [7–9]. Research continues to stress the importance of delineating mild cognitive impairment (MCI) from the prodrome of AD [9–12], while others propose that MCI might be better classified as a pre-dementia (pre-AD) condition [13–15]. In order for brief screening instruments to be effectively adapted to the primary care setting, they must be easy to interpret, accurate, and administered with only minimal supervision. In the last decade it has become clear that memory screening alone is not adequate for the early diagnosis of AD [16,17]. Differentiation of other forms of dementia with distinct neurocognitive patterns (Diffuse Lewy Body Disease, Subcortical Vascular Dementia, Frontal Lobe Dementia) from AD within patients presenting with memory complaints is of particular interest to researchers [18] as well as clinicians [19,20]. Brief screening instruments have been developed with acceptable levels of sensitivity and specificity [21–26]. However, prior studies suggest that improvements in the practical application and interpretation of these instruments will aid in their usefulness in both specialty clinics and primary care setting [7]. Brief screening instruments that provide research supported construct validity in assessing specific cognitive domains at risk are needed, specifically: orientation [27,28], visuospatial and executive processing [29–31], verbal fluency [32, 33], working memory [34–37], and attention and processing speed [38,39].

The Computerized Self Test (CST) was adapted from a paper and pencil Self Test used in the memory disorders clinic [24], which assesses all six cognitive domains as well as processing speed. The CST was designed with three important issues in mind for establishing a new cognitive screening test. First, the instrument must be constructed in such a way that the patient alone or with the assistance of a family member and/or caregiver (to assist with the computer interface only) could complete the test with minimal supervision. Second, the instrument must incorporate research findings that demonstrate that the clock drawing and verbal fluency tests are sensitive measures of early cognitive changes in dementia and AD [40,41]. Finally, the instrument must be computer and internet based to allow for easy access, to minimize professional time for administration and to facilitate objective scoring.

The CST was created following indications that assessing multiple cognitive domains within the same prediction model will aid in identifying persons at risk for developing AD [42]. The CST assesses verbal fluency, visual-spatial functions, memory, attention, executive functions, and perceptual/processing speed in approximately 15 minutes. The CST is designed to detect early deficits in one or more specific cognitive domains with adherence to the guidelines that any screening test does not produce a definitive diagnosis of dementia [43] and comprehensive neuropsychological and clinical assessments are needed to make a probable or possible diagnosis [44].

We hypothesized that the combination of measures in the CST would provide an accurate prediction model for discriminating between six experimental groups (normal, MCI, early AD, mild to moderate AD, moderate to severe AD, and severe AD) with special consideration given to the global deficits between cognitively impaired (CI) and control groups.

MATERIALS AND METHODS

Participants

This study consisted of 215 total participants with a mean age of 75.24. The 84 cognitively impaired patients (excluding patients diagnosed as MCI, $n = 27$) met all criteria set forth by NINCDS/ADRDA for the diagnosis of AD. Exclusion criteria included: stroke (large vessel), psychiatric disorders, diagnosis of alcohol abuse or alcoholism, presence of prior neurological disease, and significant sensory deficits or physical impairment that would preclude interaction with the computer or caregiver. The CI group consisted of current patients seen and followed at our memory disorders clinic that have met all criteria and received a diagnosis of AD as set forth by the National Institute of Neurological and Communicative Disorders and Stroke and the Alzheimer's disease and Related Disorders Association. Patients with MCI met appropriate criteria as outlined by Petersen [45]. The control group consisted of spouses of affected individuals and from individuals recruited from volunteer organizations working within the medical center. All controls completed the same neurocognitive procedures as the CI group with the addition of the Montreal Cognitive Assessment (MoCA) [46,47] to aid in the identification of individuals with possible mild cognitive impairments.

Table 1 shows the demographic information for each group; included in the table are the group, number in group (N), mean age, range, standard deviation (SD),

Table 1
Demographics for participants. From left to right are the diagnostic group, size, mean age, range, standard deviation, gender per group, years of education with range and standard deviation

Group	Size (N)	Mean age	Range	SD	Gender	Edu	range	SD
Control	104	75.45	58–89	7.25	M 41 F 63	15	8–20	2.70
MCI	27	67.24	53-78	6.42	M 24 F 3	14	8–20	4.07
Early AD	22	77.45	68–91	5.22	M 6 F 16	14	8–20	2.96
Mild to Moderate	33	75.21	56–94	9.08	M 14 F 19	14	12–20	3.03
Moderate to Severe	24	78.39	65–89	6.60	M 14 F 10	13	12–20	2.84
Severe	5	75.00	71–80	3.53	M 1 F 4	15	12–16	1.79

gender, and mean education in years, with range and standard deviation. The diagnosis of dementia and classification into the appropriate group (MCI, stages of dementia) were performed by an experienced Neurologist and Geriatric Psychiatrist. They had an opportunity to review the results of all cognitive data but were blinded to the results of the CST. In addition, all patients were examined and are followed either by the Neurologist or Geriatric Psychiatrist on a regular basis in the memory disorder clinic. The neurocognitive measures administered to all individuals in the memory disorders clinic are: MMSE, paper self test, Mini-Cog, test of executive functions, test of verbal fluency, MoCA (when indicated), Geriatric depression scale, caregiver/spouse/family member interview, and clinical examination. Diagnoses are based on a composite of these measures. The groups in this study were classified in a similar fashion with MMSE scores as a reference base. The MMSE scores for each group are: Control (28–30), MCI (26–29/MoCA < 26 and > 20), Early AD (23–26), mild to moderate AD (18–22), moderate to severe AD (11–18), and severe AD (< 10), respectively.

Data collection and processing

The CST was administered prior to routine neurocognitive measures given to patients in the memory disorders clinic. The patients and or caregivers were asked at the time of their appointment if they would like to participate in a research trial. All participants and or caregivers were read, signed, and agreed to the informed consent protocol approved by the Institutional Review Boards of the Volunteer Research Group and the University of Tennessee Medical Center. All participants were paid $10 for participation. The testing

procedures were carried out in a standardized fashion utilizing portable laptop computers with the patients, caregivers or both seated in examination rooms. The assessment instruments were administered in the order listed in the following section.

Assessment measures

(i) The CST is internet based and takes approximately 15 minutes to complete. It provides a user friendly interface with both written and oral instructions. If the participant reports experience with computers, he or she continues on with the test independently. If the participant reports no experience with computers and requires help to operate a computer, the caregiver is asked to administer the test. Alternatively, if asked, a technician is also available for assistance with test administration. The caregiver, family member, or technician may manipulate the mouse or arrows for the patient or facilitate the typing and entering of patient responses. These individuals, however, are given explicit instructions not to provide aid or hints to the patient in order to obtain the most accurate results. The CST was not used in the diagnostic criteria for any of the study participants. The CST was created with carefully manipulated assessment and scoring mechanisms that are unique to this instrument. In cognitive testing, there is often significant overlap between test content [48], in part due to the inherent nature of human cognition and its dependence on language. Thus, in content, scoring, and delivery, the CST is a novel and unique instrument. Painstaking attention was also applied to the results as seen by the patient, such that no inference or indication that may lead to the interpretation of a diagnosis of dementia is given to the patient.

CST content

The CST obtains demographic information on the initial screen. This information includes, gender, age, computer experience, self-report of memory problems, family history of memory problems or dementia and if assistance is needed to complete the CST. The CST assesses six cognitive domains.

Visual spatial/executive processing

The clock drawing test [49,50] is presented on three screens. First the participant is presented a selection of four geometric shapes from which he or she is to choose the shape that best represents a clock face. Second, clock numbers (12, 3, 6, and 9) are presented in succession. The participant is asked to click on the clock face where each of the numbers should go. Finally, the participant is presented a selection of clock hands. Only one clock-hand set will produce the time at ten after eleven. The participant has to click on the correct choice and can score up to 4 points. This type of clock construction task reduces the demand on motoric functions [51] and reduces the likelihood of errors in scoring due to motor slowing produced in normal aging [52].

Working memory

Engle and colleagues [53] proposed that working memory [54–56] capacity is the ability to temporarily maintain representations with distraction or interference. The complex span task requires maintenance of a list of items to be recalled in the face of other information that needs to be processed but is irrelevant to the memory task. Hence, list elements must be maintained in working memory, but in addition, the task requires executive attention [57,58] in order to preserve these representations during an interference or secondary task. The memory and attention subtests were developed with these fundamental concepts in mind. The participants are presented three words and given instructions to study the words and commit them to memory. The participants are then presented a screen with three blank text boxes after the verbal fluency section of the test and asked to type in the three words. The memory section algorithm automatically detects the correct word based on the first three letters and it is entered into the text field for the patient. There are 3 points possible for this section. The three words

for the memory subtest are maintained algorithmically and randomly changed for each test administration to hinder possible test-retest learning effects.

Verbal fluency

Verbal fluency has been demonstrated to be an important component of semantic memory. The verbal fluency section of the CST asks participants to name 15 animals as quickly as possible. The database for verbal fluency operates through an algorithm of word-pattern matching (includes ~2,000 animal names) such that when the first three or four letters are identified, the computer automatically completes the word and enters it into the text space; therefore, the patients are not penalized points for spelling. Similarly, perseverative effects are controlled for such that repeated words are not rewarded. There are a total of 15 points possible for this section.

Attention

The attention section reflects components as described by Engle [53] such that the participants are asked to type in the names of 5 months prior to December in reverse order (e.g., December, November, October). This test maintains active engagement of working memory, attention, and concept organization. Like the other text entry subtests, the first three or four letters are automatically detected and entered. Spelling does not affect the total points for this section. There are a total of 5 points in this section.

Orientation

The participants are asked to recall the current year, current month, and current date. The auto-detection feature is also present in this section. There are a total of 3 points for this section.

Processing speed

The time or processing speed is used for comparison to control samples and statistical classification – patients are not penalized for the total time. Time is measured for each subtest and for the total time of completion. Patients are advised that it is a timed test and are encouraged to complete it as quickly and accurately as possible. To prevent extraordinary amounts of time being used by non-interaction with the test, after 30 seconds of inactivation (e.g., no mouse or keyboard movement), the test will automatically progress to the next screen. Hence, inactivity will result in sections being missed thereby lowering the total score.

User interface

The CST provides a user friendly interface and is easily manipulated with rudimentary computer skills. In our sample, the technician remained in the room with patient and or patient/caregiver for the entire test completion in order to passively monitor compliance, interactions, and record behavioral observations. Behavioral Rating Scales (BRS) were created for the technician to record observations and the severity of behavioral and psychiatric symptoms and functional ability. The BRS consist of a five point rating system 1 = no problems or difficulty and 5 = severe problems and difficulty. The ratings consist of orientation, motor functions, attention, and retention of task, comprehension, and awareness of task. In addition, the BRS recorded any attempts by the caregiver/or family member who were assisting the patient with the computer interface to improve the patient's score.

(ii) Mini Mental State Examination (MMSE) [59] (MiniMental, LLC): The MMSE is probably the most widely used test of cognitive function. It is extensively used as a screening tool in the diagnosis of dementia as well as to assess severity and change over time. The MMSE has a maximum score of 30 points. The test items are orientation to time and place (10 points), registration of 3 words (3), attention and calculation (5), recall of 3 words (3), language (8) and visual construction (1).

(iii) Executive Functions: The written test of executive functions is routinely administered to patients in the memory disorders clinic. This test assesses concept formation, attention, self-monitoring and reasoning for abstract concepts, including proverbs and similarities [60]. It also presents three abstract concepts: How much does an elephant weigh? How many camels are in California? An abstract maze problem is given – a blank rectangle is presented with a problem: I have lost my keys on a football field, show me how you would search for them. Self monitoring, attention and self regulation are assessed by finger tapping tests [61]. The total possible score is 15 points.

(iv) Verbal Fluency: The test of verbal fluency contains three sections, each 1 minute in length. The participants are asked to recall as many animals + vegetables + fruits as possible within the allotted time. The cut-off for abnormal performance is < 38 (total).

(v) Mini-Cog: The Mini-Cog test is freely downloadable from http://www.hospitalmedicine.org /geriresource/toolbox/welcome.htm. It is a 3-minute instrument used to screen for cognitive impairment in older adults. It utilizes a three-item recall test for memory screening and a simply scored version of the clock drawing test serving as interference for the working memory task. The Mini-Cog was administered and scored utilizing the standard procedures in [62].

(vi) Geriatric Depression Scale (GDS): The Geriatric Depression Scale (GDS) is one of the most commonly used depression screening instruments in elderly populations. The scale is a 30 item, easily administer inventory that has been used widely to assess elderly populations in communities and institutions, including hospitals and nursing homes [63–66].

Data analysis

Discriminant Analysis was employed to determine the accuracy of the CST, MMSE, and Mini-Cog in the classification of cognitively impaired and control groups and in classification of the six groups in this study. Discriminant analysis builds a predictive model for group membership, which is composed of a set of discriminant functions based on linear combinations of the predictor variables that provide the superlative discrimination between the groups. We elected discriminant analysis based on its robustness despite modest violations to the assumptions of normality [67]. Procedures, however, typically violating multivariate normality (e.g., dichotomous variables) are not likely to affect conclusions based on discriminant analysis [68]. Reliability and validity analyses were conducted for the obtained scores on the CST comparing them to subtest scores on the MMSE, Mini-Cog, the paper version of the CST, and the written and administered versions of verbal fluency and executive functions. We compared the means between cognitively impaired and controls for demographic variables and total test scores not assuming equal variances. We then performed a test-retest analysis for 38 CI patients and 10 controls at ~six weeks. For this analysis we utilized a two-way random effects model with an absolute agreement definition and the Pearson product-moment correlation coefficient. Multivariate analysis of variance (MANOVA) was utilized to compare the diagnostic groups to determine significant differences for each diagnostic group compared to controls for the CST. The mean difference was compared using the Tukey adjustment with alpha=0.05.

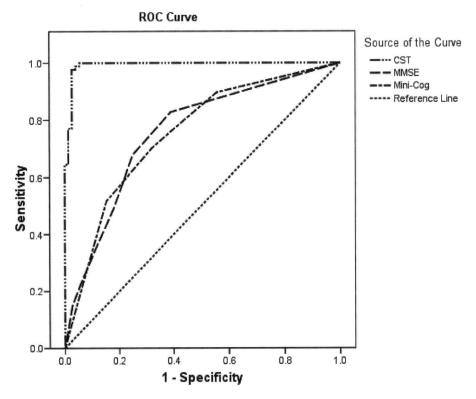

Fig. 1. ROC illustrating sensitivity and specificity of the CST, MMSE, and Mini-Cog for detection of cognitive impairment with MMSE cutoff at 24.

RESULTS

Accuracy, sensitivity, and specificity

The discriminant analysis results show the CST correctly classified 91% of the six experimental groups listed in Table 1, and 96% of the two groups (cognitively impaired and control). The MMSE correctly classified 54% of the six groups and 71% of the two groups. The Mini-Cog correctly classified 48% of the six groups and 69% of the two groups. The probabilities for group inclusion (normal/CI) from the discriminant analysis with the cutoff set at MMSE = 24 were entered into a receiver-operating characteristic curve (ROC) analysis. The CST area under the curve (AUC) is 99%, SE (0.006), p (0.000), with sensitivity of 99% and specificity of 95%. The MMSE AUC is 82% SE (0.039), p (0.000) with sensitivity at 83% and specificity of 38%. The Mini-Cog AUC is 89% SE (0.039), p (0.000) with sensitivity at 89% and specificity of 55%. Figure 1 shows the ROC curves for each of the measures.

Reliability and validity

The total score for the CST is positively correlated with the total score on the MMSE, $r = 0.56, p < 0.000$. The CST orientation subtest shows significant correlations with the orientation to time ($r = 0.79, p < 0.000$) and place ($r = 0.66, p < 0.000$) of the MMSE. The working memory subtest for the CST is correlated with the recall test of the MMSE at significant levels ($r = 0.61, p < 0.000$). The test of attention for the CST is correlated with the test of attention on the MMSE ($r = 0.69, p < 0.000$). The verbal fluency subtest on the CST is correlated with test of verbal fluency ($r = 0.53, p < 0.000$). Similarly the clock subtest is correlated with tests of executive functions ($r = 0.35, p = 0.003$) and the intersecting pentagons subtest on MMSE ($r = 0.36, p = 0.018$). We assessed reliability using a two-way random effects model with an internal consistency definition. The intra-class correlations (ICC) for the CST orientation subtest and MMSE orientation to both place and time are 0.72 for single measures and 0.88 for average measures ($p < 0.00$). The CST total

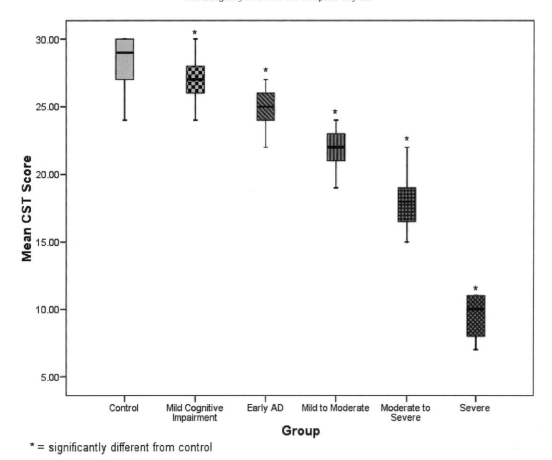

Fig. 2. MANOVA results for mean CST scores for each of the diagnostic groups compared to controls.

* = significantly different from control

score and scores on tests of executive functions (e.g., proverbs, finger tapping, similarities) show (ICC) of 0.43 for single measures and 0.61 for average measures ($p < 0.00$). The memory subtest on CST and recall on MMSE show an ICC of 0.61 for single measures and 0.76 for average measures ($p < 0.00$). The attention subtests on CST and MMSE show ICC of 0.27 for single measures and 0.43 for average measures ($p = 0.04$). The correlation between the CST and the paper version is 0.98, ($p < 0.01$), similar results are shown for the internal consistency analysis between the CST and paper version (17) with an average measure of 0.98, F (155.13), $p < 0.000$. The CST memory subtest shows a positive correlation to the total of the Mini-Cog 0.71 ($p < 0.000$), as does the total clock for CST 0.28, ($p < 0.000$). The test-retest for the total group of 48 at ~six weeks produces a Chronbach's alpha of 0.76 with F (47) = 4.17, $p < 0.00$.

Multivariate tests between diagnostic groups

The means for the CST for each diagnostic group are plotted in Fig. 2. On the y axis is the mean CST score and on the x axis are the diagnostic groups. The MANOVA results show the differences for each group compared to controls are significant. The MCI mean 26.96, SD=1.63, Mean difference (MD)=1.43*, and standard error (SE)=0.33. The early AD group mean is 24.77, SD=1.31, MD=3.62*, SE=0.362. The Mild to moderate group mean is 22.03, SD=1.49, MD=6.86*, SE=0.308. The moderate to severe group mean is 17.83, SD=1.83, MD=10.56*, SE=0.349. The severe group mean is 9.4, SD=1.82, MD=18.99*, SE=0.706. The asterisk indicates significant at < 0.01.

Table 2 shows the results for the univariate tests for the MANOVA procedure. In the table from left to right are the dependent variable, sum of squares, degrees of

Table 2

Univariate tests for the MANOVA procedures. From left to right are demographic, self report and cognitive measures, the sum of squares and error, degrees of freedom, mean square, F for the test, significance, partial eta squared, and the observed power. Each of the dependent variables is significant when the diagnostic groups is a between subject factor. The partial eta (effect size) shows that the CST accounts for 89% of the variance between the groups in this study. The observed power indicates the sample size is adequate for the statistical procedures utilized

Dependent variable		Sum of squares	df	Mean square	F	Sig	Partial eta squared	Observed power (a)
CST	Corthast	4030.769	5	806.154	338.893	0.000	0.890	1.000
	Error	497.166	209	2.379				
SRMP	Corthast	14.448	5	2.890	15.610	0.000	0.272	1.000
	Error	38.687	209	0.185				
FM HX	Corthast	4.321	5	0.864	4.115	0.001	0.090	0.953
	Error	43.893	209	0.210				
GENDER	Corthast	6.928	5	1.386	6.219	0.000	0.130	0.996
	Error	46.561	209	0.223				
AGE	Corthast	1270.146	5	254.029	4.881	0.000	0.105	0.980
	Error	10878.412	209	52.050				
CSTTIME	Corthast	220.380	5	44.076	3.969	0.002	0.087	0.945
	Error	2320.705	209	11.104				
MINI-COG	Corthast	83.695	5	16.739	15.266	0.000	0.268	1.000
	Error	229.161	209	1.096				
MMSE	Corthast	1886.741	5	377.348	37.573	0.000	0.480	1.000
	Error	2044.580	209	9.783				

freedom, mean square, F value, significance level, partial eta squared (the proportion of the effect + error variance that is attributable to the effect), and the observed power (or adequacy of the sample size for the statistical procedure). The mean time for completion of the CST in minutes and seconds is $\leqslant 6.10$ for controls, 7.5 for MCI, 8.11 for early AD, 8.57 for mild to moderate, and $\geqslant 9.00$ for both moderate to severe and severe. Clinical observations suggest that if the patient takes longer than 13 minutes to complete the CST, the score will not improve. Similarly, the more severe groups may finish the CST in as little as 3 minutes due to the inability to complete the items.

The results of the t-tests between CI and controls for all behavioral ratings (BRS) show the CI group exhibits more difficulties in orientation t (5.48), $p < 0.000$, motor functions t (3.65), $p < 0.000$, attention t (6.02), $p < 0.000$, task comprehension t (3.97), $p < 0.000$, task retention t (6.23), $p < 0.000$. The CI group had significantly more caregiver assisted administration than controls t (6.78), $p < 0.000$. Of interest the CI group reported more computer literacy than controls with t (5.76), $p < 0.000$) (possibly associated with anosoagnosia). The degree of difficulty with self administration increases relative to the stage of the disease. Thus far, the data indicate that the caregiver assisted administration did not affect the accuracy of the discriminant classification.

DISCUSSION

The CST provides an alternative to traditional paper based methods for assessing neurobehavioral and cog-

nitive functions. The individual may complete the CST alone or receive assistance from a caregiver or other non-professional acting only to facilitate the computer interface. The current data indicate that the CST is a valid and sensitive instrument for evaluating functional deficits in both global and specific cognitive domains. The total CST score, processing speed (time to complete the CST), self-report of memory problems, age, family history of AD, and gender offer a reliable and accurate prediction model for classifying and discriminating between normal, MCI, and various stages within AD for the population in our study. Recent data suggests that 21% of a multiethnic group of normal elderly subjects progressed to MCI at a rate of 5% per year. For those individuals presenting initially with MCI, 22% were subsequently diagnosed with AD at a rate of 5% per year [69]. 47% of the cohort remained unchanged and a rather large number (31%) reverted to normal. Individuals with MCI that had impairments in memory and at least one other cognitive domain were shown to be highly associated with greatest risk for conversion to AD and these patients were less likely to revert to normal at follow-up [69]. In addition, research has shown that AD patients may show cognitive deficits many years prior to the diagnosis of dementia [70,71].

The CST shows a high rate of successfully classifying global cognitive impairment from normal cognitive functioning and does so with significant accuracy, sensitivity, and specificity with the consideration that increased sample size does increase the additive property of screening tests [48]. The current findings are important for populations exhibiting early symptoms of

MCI as well as those individuals that have a family history of AD. Early computerized cognitive monitoring may prove important for both populations exhibiting early functional symptoms as well as those individuals that have a family history of AD. In addition, as the population ages many individuals become increasingly concerned about their own cognitive health (i.e., the worried well) [72].

The CST provides an easily interpreted and administered method of obtaining a baseline of cognitive functioning. One of the primary objectives for the CST is to increase the likelihood of detecting the earliest declines in cognitive functioning in order to decrease the number of individuals that go undiagnosed in the primary care setting. However, with the development of any screening test, expressed consideration needs to be given to reducing the likelihood of a misdiagnosis or false positive. The CST does not provide any diagnostic information to the patient in the results section. Painstaking effort was put into the wording and presentation of deficits such that the likelihood of an interpretation of dementia from the results is minimized. The benefits of correct detection of deficits for the patient include the implementation of more extensive assessment and testing procedures to accurately diagnose the syndrome and initiation of medications that have been shown to produce positive benefits [4]. The harm due to false positive results involves not only the cost of further testing but also the emotional effects on the patient. These issues are discussed in more detail in a recent review [48].

If the data obtained in this early study continues to demonstrate, as larger samples become available, a distinct pattern of variable cognitive changes in MCI and stages of AD an emerging concept of a domain specific cognitive patterns (DSCP) may continue to develop. This concept may offer a novel and important direction for further research. It will be possible to construct large data sets for standardizing DSCP in order to identify deficits and classify individual patients more quickly and accurately.

The CST, in the current population, is sensitive to differences between normal, MCI, and stages within AD by assessing functionality in six cognitive domains (memory, verbal fluency, orientation, visuospatial organization, executive function, and attention). The MANOVA results show there are significant deficits for the CI group as compared to controls. The effect size for the CST accounts for 89% of the variance between all diagnostic groups. Additionally, the variables included in the discriminant function appear to provide an accurate predictive model. However, future research will include additional cognitive modules and intensive analysis of the functional relationships between cognitive component-processes.

Several additions may strengthen the current study. It is inherently true that any screening instrument will perform more efficiently in predefined groups as opposed to consecutive or unknown populations. Further analysis of concurrent validity with other widely used cognitive screening instruments (MoCA, Dementia Rating Scale, WAIS memory scale) is desirable. Recent research suggests that practice effects are evident for some of the tasks in the CogState battery [73]. We would also like to obtain large samples of ethnic and culturally diverse populations for further study and standardization. The population in this study is from one local center with mostly Caucasian individuals with a high degree of the patients being well-educated; therefore, larger samples are needed. These limitations will continue to be addressed as our research continues. The CST utilizes variations of substantiated neurocognitive assessment procedures and further additions are planned. Additionally, upon the completion of more clinical trials and independent validation the discriminant functions will be available via internet access for physicians to determine the probability of inclusion in specific diagnostic groups based on the patient's individual domain specific cognitive profile. The results of the discriminant analysis will provide the specific probability of inclusion into specific diagnostic groups. All patients in this study are followed in the memory disorders clinic and we will continue to obtain longitudinal data. This system of testing will continue to develop and we will be incorporating other clinical populations (i.e., non-amnestic and non-AD dementia types) in future studies.

ACKNOWLEDGMENTS

The authors would like to express sincere gratitude to Dr. Richard Gibson, A.D. Baxter and Libby Hall for their contributions and conscientious effort in the memory disorders clinic. The authors express sincere gratitude to Charles Licata and Mateja de Leonni Stanonik for their dedicated work in the development of the paper self test. The authors also would like to thank the patients, family members and volunteers that participated in this study.

Authors' disclosures available online (http://www.j-alz.com/disclosures/view.php?id=232).

REFERENCES

[1] Flaks MK, Yassuda MS, Regina AC, Cid CG, Camargo CH, Gattaz WF, Forlenza OV (2006) The Short Cognitive Performance Test (SKT): a preliminary study of its psychometric properties in Brazil. *Int Psychogeriatr* **18**, 121-133.

[2] Kalbe E, Salmon E, Perani D, Holthoff V, Sorbi S, Elsner A, Weisenbach S, Brand M, Lenz O, Kessler J, Luedecke S, Ortelli P, Herholz K (2005) Anosognosia in very mild Alzheimer's disease but not in mild cognitive impairment. *Dement Geriatr Cogn Disord* **19**, 349-356.

[3] Cullen B, O'Neill B, Evans JJ, Coen RF, Lawlor BA (2007) A review of screening tests for cognitive impairment. *J Neurol Neurosurg Psychiatry* **78**, 790-799.

[4] Tinklenberg JR, Kraemer HC, Yaffe K, Ross L, Sheikh J, Ashford JW, Yesavage JA, Taylor JL (2007) Donepezil treatment and Alzheimer disease: can the results of randomized clinical trials be applied to Alzheimer disease patients in clinical practice? *Am J Geriatr Psychiatry* **15**, 953-960.

[5] Petersen RC, Thomas RG, Grundman M, Bennett D, Doody R, Ferris S, Galasko D, Jin S, Kaye J, Levey A, Pfeiffer E, Sano M, van Dyck CH, Thal LJ (2005) Vitamin E and donepezil for the treatment of mild cognitive impairment. *N Engl J Med* **352**, 2379-2388.

[6] Knopman DS (2006) Current treatment of mild cognitive impairment and Alzheimer's disease. *Curr Neurol Neurosci Rep* **6**, 365-371.

[7] Evans R ed. (1999) *Diagnostic Testing in Neurology*, W.B. Saunders, Philadelphia.

[8] Ashford JW, Borson S (2008) Primary care screening for dementia and mild cognitive impairment. *JAMA* **299**, 1132-1133; author reply 1133-1134.

[9] Ashford JW, Borson S, O'Hara R, Dash P, Frank L, Robert P, Shankle WR, Tierney M, Brody H, Schmitt FA, Kraemer HC, Buschke H, Fillit H (2007) Should older adults be screened for dementia? It is important to screen for evidence of dementia! *Alzheimers Dement* **3**, 75-80.

[10] Petersen RC, Bennett D (2005) Mild cognitive impairment: is it Alzheimer's disease or not? *J Alzheimers Dis* **7**, 241-245; discussion 255-262.

[11] Petersen RC, Morris JC (2005) Mild cognitive impairment as a clinical entity and treatment target. *Arch Neurol* **62**, 1160-1163; discussion 1167.

[12] Petersen RC, Smith GE, Waring SC, Ivnik RJ, Tangalos EG, Kokmen E (1999) Mild cognitive impairment: clinical characterization and outcome. *Arch Neurol* **56**, 303-308.

[13] Flicker C, Ferris SH, Reisberg B (1991) Mild cognitive impairment in the elderly: predictors of dementia. *Neurology* **41**, 1006-1009.

[14] Morris JC, Cummings J (2005) Mild cognitive impairment (MCI) represents early-stage Alzheimer's disease. *J Alzheimers Dis* **7**, 235-239; discussion 255-262.

[15] Yesavage JA, O'Hara R, Kraemer H, Noda A, Taylor JL, Ferris S, Gely-Nargeot MC, Rosen A, Friedman L, Sheikh J, Derouesne C (2002) Modeling the prevalence and incidence of Alzheimer's disease and mild cognitive impairment. *J Psychiatr Res* **36**, 281-286.

[16] Hofman M, Seifritz E, Krauchi K, Hock C, Hampel H, Neugebauer A, Muller-Spahn F (2000) Alzheimer's disease, depression and normal ageing: merit of simple psychomotor and visuospatial tasks. *Int J Geriatr Psychiatry* **15**, 31-39.

[17] Kinjo H (2007) Improving sensitivity of the recognition task in the Alzheimer's Disease Assessment Scale. *Psychol Rep* **100**, 420-426.

[18] Kilada S, Gamaldo A, Grant EA, Moghekar A, Morris JC, O'Brien RJ (2005) Brief screening tests for the diagnosis of dementia: comparison with the mini-mental state exam. *Alzheimer Dis Assoc Disord* **19**, 8-16.

[19] Knopman DS (1998) Current pharmacotherapies for Alzheimer's disease. *Geriatrics* **53 Suppl 1**, S31-34.

[20] Trenkle DL, Shankle WR, Azen SP (2007) Detecting cognitive impairment in primary care: performance assessment of three screening instruments. *J Alzheimers Dis* **11**, 323-335.

[21] Brown J, Pengas G, Dawson K, Brown LA, Clatworthy P (2009) Self administered cognitive screening test (TYM) for detection of Alzheimer's disease: cross sectional study. *BMJ* **338**, b2030.

[22] De Jager CA, Hogervorst E, Combrinck M, Budge MM (2003) Sensitivity and specificity of neuropsychological tests for mild cognitive impairment, vascular cognitive impairment and Alzheimer's disease. *Psychol Med* **33**, 1039-1050.

[23] de Jager CA, Schrijnemaekers AC, Honey TE, Budge MM (2009) Detection of MCI in the clinic: evaluation of the sensitivity and specificity of a computerised test battery, the Hopkins Verbal Learning Test and the MMSE. *Age Ageing* **38**, 455-460.

[24] de Leonni Stanonik M, Licata CA, Walton NC, Lounsbury JW, Hutson RK, Dougherty JH, Jr. (2005) The Self Test: a screening tool for dementia requiring minimal supervision. *Int Psychogeriatr* **17**, 669-678.

[25] Saxton J, Morrow L, Eschman A, Archer G, Luther J, Zuccolotto A (2009) Computer assessment of mild cognitive impairment. *Postgrad Med* **121**, 177-185.

[26] Saxton J, Snitz BE, Lopez OL, Ives DG, Dunn LO, Fitzpatrick A, Carlson MC, Dekosky ST (2009) Functional and cognitive criteria produce different rates of mild cognitive impairment and conversion to dementia. *J Neurol Neurosurg Psychiatry* **80**, 737-743.

[27] Kalman J, Magloczky E, Janka Z (1995) Disturbed visuospatial orientation in the early stage of Alzheimer's dementia. *Arch Gerontol Geriatr* **21**, 27-34.

[28] Wright M, Geffen G, Geffen L (1997) Comparative effects of ageing and dementia of the Alzheimer type on orientation of visual attention. *Dement Geriatr Cogn Disord* **8**, 366-375.

[29] Borson S, Brush M, Gil E, Scanlan J, Vitaliano P, Chen J, Cashman J, Sta Maria MM, Barnhart R, Roques J (1999) The Clock Drawing Test: utility for dementia detection in multiethnic elders. *J Gerontol A Biol Sci Med Sci* **54**, M534-540.

[30] Heinik J, Solomesh I, Shein V, Becker D (2002) Clock drawing test in mild and moderate dementia of the Alzheimer's type: a comparative and correlation study. *Int J Geriatr Psychiatry* **17**, 480-485.

[31] Schramm U, Berger G, Muller R, Kratzsch T, Peters J, Frolich L (2002) Psychometric properties of Clock Drawing Test and MMSE or Short Performance Test (SKT) in dementia screening in a memory clinic population. *Int J Geriatr Psychiatry* **17**, 254-260.

[32] Cummings JL (2004) The one-minute mental status examination. *Neurology* **62**, 534-535.

[33] Murphy KJ, Rich JB, Troyer AK (2006) Verbal fluency patterns in amnestic mild cognitive impairment are characteristic of Alzheimer's type dementia. *J Int Neuropsychol Soc* **12**, 570-574.

[34] Backman L (2008) Memory and cognition in preclinical dementia: what we know and what we do not know. *Can J Psychiatry* **53**, 354-360.

[35] Backman L, Jones S, Berger AK, Laukka EJ, Small BJ (2005) Cognitive impairment in preclinical Alzheimer's disease: a meta-analysis. *Neuropsychology* **19**, 520-531.

[36] Barnes LL, Schneider JA, Boyle PA, Bienias JL, Bennett DA (2006) Memory complaints are related to Alzheimer disease pathology in older persons. *Neurology* **67**, 1581-1585.

[37] Sambataro F, Murty VP, Callicott JH, Tan HY, Das S, Weinberger DR, Mattay VS (2008) Age-related alterations in default mode network: Impact on working memory performance. *Neurobiol Aging*, in press.

[38] Pereira FS, Yassuda MS, Oliveira AM, Forlenza OV (2008) Executive dysfunction correlates with impaired functional status in older adults with varying degrees of cognitive impairment. *Int Psychogeriatr*, 1-12.

[39] Traykov L, Raoux N, Latour F, Gallo L, Hanon O, Baudic S, Bayle C, Wenisch E, Remy P, Rigaud AS (2007) Executive functions deficit in mild cognitive impairment. *Cogn Behav Neurol* **20**, 219-224.

[40] Thomann PA, Toro P, Dos Santos V, Essig M, Schroder J (2008) Clock drawing performance and brain morphology in mild cognitive impairment and Alzheimer's disease. *Brain Cogn* **67**, 88-93.

[41] Zhou Y, Dougherty JH, Jr., Hubner KF, Bai B, Cannon RL, Hutson RK (2008) Abnormal connectivity in the posterior cingulate and hippocampus in early Alzheimer's disease and mild cognitive impairment. *Alzheimers Dement* **4**, 265-270.

[42] Backman L, Jones S, Berger AK, Laukka EJ, Small BJ (2004) Multiple cognitive deficits during the transition to Alzheimer's disease. *J Intern Med* **256**, 195-204.

[43] American Psychiatric Association (2000) Diagnostic and statistical manual of mental disorders (4th ed., text revision). Washington, DC.

[44] (1998) Guidelines for the evaluation of dementia and age-related cognitive decline. American Psychological Association Presidential Task Force. *Am Psychol* **53**, 1298-1303.

[45] Petersen RC (2004) Mild cognitive impairment as a diagnostic entity. *J Intern Med* **256**, 183-194.

[46] Nasreddine ZS, Phillips NA, Bedirian V, Charbonneau S, Whitehead V, Collin I, Cummings JL, Chertkow H (2005) The Montreal Cognitive Assessment, MoCA: a brief screening tool for mild cognitive impairment. *J Am Geriatr Soc* **53**, 695-699.

[47] Olson RA, Chhanabhai T, McKenzie M (2008) Feasibility study of the Montreal Cognitive Assessment (MoCA) in patients with brain metastases. *Support Care Cancer* **16**, 1273-1278.

[48] Ashford AE (2008) Screening for memory disorders, dementia and Alzheimer's disease. *Aging Health* **4**, 399-432.

[49] Cahn DA, Salmon DP, Monsch AU, Butters N, Wiederholt WC, Corey-Bloom J, Barrett-Connor E (1996) Screening for dementia of the alzheimer type in the community: the utility of the Clock Drawing Test. *Arch Clin Neuropsychol* **11**, 529-539.

[50] Lessig MC, Scanlan JM, Nazemi H, Borson S (2008) Time that tells: critical clock-drawing errors for dementia screening. *Int Psychogeriatr* **20**, 459-470.

[51] Raz N, Rodrigue KM (2006) Differential aging of the brain: patterns, cognitive correlates and modifiers. *Neurosci Biobehav Rev* **30**, 730-748.

[52] Cosentino S, Jefferson A, Chute DL, Kaplan E, Libon DJ (2004) Clock drawing errors in dementia: neuropsychological and neuroanatomical considerations. *Cogn Behav Neurol* **17**, 74-84.

[53] Engle RW, Tuholski SW, Laughlin JE, Conway AR (1999) Working memory, short-term memory, and general fluid intelligence: a latent-variable approach. *J Exp Psychol Gen* **128**, 309-331.

[54] Baddeley A, Hitch GJL (1974) *Working Memory. in The psychology of learning and motivation: advances in research and theory*, Academic Press, New York.

[55] Baddeley A, Cocchini G, Della Sala S, Logie RH, Spinnler H (1999) Working memory and vigilance: evidence from normal aging and Alzheimer's disease. *Brain Cogn* **41**, 87-108.

[56] Baddeley AD, Bressi S, Della Sala S, Logie R, Spinnler H (1991) The decline of working memory in Alzheimer's disease. A longitudinal study. *Brain* **114** (Pt 6), 2521-2542.

[57] Cannon R, Congedo, M, Lubar, J., Hutchens, T. (2009) Differentiating at network of executive attention: LORETA Neurofeedback in anterior cingulate and dorsolateral prefrontal cortices. *Int J Neurosci* **119**, 404-441.

[58] Cannon R, Lubar J, Congedo M, Thornton K, Towler K, Hutchens T (2007) The effects of neurofeedback training in the cognitive division of the anterior cingulate gyrus. *Int J Neurosci* **117**, 337-357.

[59] Folstein MF, Folstein SE, McHugh PR (1975) "Mini-mental state". A practical method for grading the cognitive state of patients for the clinician. *J Psychiatr Res* **12**, 189-198.

[60] Lafleche GaMSA (1995) Executive Function Deficits in Mild Alzheimer's Disease. *Neuropsychology* **9**, 313-320.

[61] Prigatano GP, Johnson SC, Gale SD (2004) Neuroimaging correlates of the Halstead Finger Tapping Test several years post-traumatic brain injury. *Brain Inj* **18**, 661-669.

[62] Borson S, Scanlan J, Brush M, Vitaliano P, Dokmak A (2000) The mini-cog: a cognitive 'vital signs' measure for dementia screening in multi-lingual elderly. *Int J Geriatr Psychiatry* **15**, 1021-1027.

[63] Yesavage J (1993) Differential diagnosis between depression and dementia. *Am J Med* **94**, 23S-28S.

[64] Yesavage JA (1991) Geriatric depression scale: consistency of depressive symptoms over time. *Percept Mot Skills* **73**, 1032.

[65] Yesavage JA (1988) Geriatric Depression Scale. *Psychopharmacol Bull* **24**, 709-711.

[66] Yesavage JA, Brink TL, Rose TL, Lum O, Huang V, Adey M, Leirer VO (1982) Development and validation of a geriatric depression screening scale: a preliminary report. *J Psychiatr Res* **17**, 37-49.

[67] Lachenbruch PA (1975) Discriminant Analysis. *Biometrics* **35**, 69-85.

[68] Klecka WR (1980) *Discriminant Analysis*, Sage Publications, Beverly Hills.

[69] Manly JJ, Tang MX, Schupf N, Stern Y, Vonsattel JP, Mayeux R (2008) Frequency and course of mild cognitive impairment in a multiethnic community. *Ann Neurol* **63**, 494-506.

[70] Kemper S, Marquis J, Thompson M (2001) Longitudinal change in language production: effects of aging and dementia on grammatical complexity and propositional content. *Psychol Aging* **16**, 600-614.

[71] La Rue A, Jarvik LF (1987) Cognitive function and prediction of dementia in old age. *Int J Aging Hum Dev* **25**, 79-89.

[72] Ahmed S, Mitchell J, Arnold R, Dawson K, Nestor PJ, Hodges JR (2008) Memory complaints in mild cognitive impairment, worried well, and semantic dementia patients. *Alzheimer Dis Assoc Disord* **22**, 227-235.

[73] Falleti MG, Maruff P, Collie A, Darby DG (2006) Practice effects associated with the repeated assessment of cognitive function using the CogState battery at 10-minute, one week and one month test-retest intervals. *J Clin Exp Neuropsychol* **28**, 1095-1112.

Praise for COGselftest

I use the CST in my clinical practice as a tool to help differentiate between dementia subtypes and monitor cognitive status over time. It is imperative to correctly identify and diagnose each patient so that resources can be tailored to provide the best possible care.

— **Dr. Monica Crane**
Neurologist
Knoxville, Tennessee

Providing innovative, quality disease screening and diagnostic services to our patients is a priority for the Summit Medical Group. As the first major primary care provider organization to offer this test, Summit continues to deliver on that priority. We are impressed with the quality and depth of information that the COGselftest results provide our physicians as well as the ease-of-use of the test. We look forward to making a difference in the fight against Alzheimer's and related dementias.

— **Jack Kam**
Vice President
Ancillary Services and Business Development
Summit Medical Group

Nobody that I've come across is really afraid of the test and I think that's important. They don't feel alienated by it and are comfortable taking it. It speaks to the individual taking the test with verbal instructions.

— **Rex Cannon**
Researcher
University of Tennessee, Knoxville

Made in the USA
Charleston, SC
04 April 2015